THE HAND

Anatomy, Examination, and Diagnosis

Editors
Ghazi Rayan, MD
Edward Akelman, MD

Contributors and Publications and Products Advisory Committee (PPAC) members

Richard Bernstein, MD
Jeffrey Budoff, MD
Charles Goldfarb, MD
Thomas Hughes, MD
Steven L. Peterson, MD
Craig Phillips, MD
Jay Pomerance, MD
Matthew Putnam, MD
Jennifer Wolf, MD

THE HAND
Anatomy, Examination, and Diagnosis

AMERICAN SOCIETY FOR SURGERY OF THE HAND

Fourth Edition

ASSH

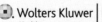 Wolters Kluwer | Lippincott Williams & Wilkins
Health

Philadelphia · Baltimore · New York · London
Buenos Aires · Hong Kong · Sydney · Tokyo

Acquisitions Editor: Robert Hurley
Product Manager: Elise M. Paxson
Production Manager: Bridgett Dougherty
Senior Manufacturing Manager: Benjamin Rivera
Marketing Manager: Lisa Lawrence
Design Coordinator: Doug Smock
Production Service: Aptara, Inc.

LIPPINCOTT WILLIAMS & WILKINS, a WOLTERS KLUWER business
Two Commerce Square
2001 Market Street
Philadelphia, PA 19103 USA
LWW.com

Printed in China

Library of Congress Cataloging-in-Publication Data

ISBN number: 978-1-45111-593-2
CIP data available upon request

© The American Society for Surgery of the Hand, 2011, 1990, 1983, 1978

Care has been taken to confirm the accuracy of the information presented and to describe generally accepted practices. However, the authors, editors, and publisher are not responsible for errors or omissions or for any consequences from application of the information in this book and make no warranty, expressed or implied, with respect to the currency, completeness, or accuracy of the contents of the publication. Application of the information in a particular situation remains the professional responsibility of the practitioner.

The authors, editors, and publisher have exerted every effort to ensure that drug selection and dosage set forth in this text are in accordance with current recommendations and practice at the time of publication. However, in view of ongoing research, changes in government regulations, and the constant flow of information relating to drug therapy and drug reactions, the reader is urged to check the package insert for each drug for any change in indications and dosage and for added warnings and precautions. This is particularly important when the recommended agent is a new or infrequently employed drug.

Some drugs and medical devices presented in the publication have Food and Drug Administration (FDA) clearance for limited use in restricted research settings. It is the responsibility of the health care provider to ascertain the FDA status of each drug or device planned for use in their clinical practice.

To purchase additional copies of this book, call our customer service department at (800) 638–3030 or fax orders to (301) 223–2320. International customers should call (301) 223–2300.

Visit Lippincott Williams & Wilkins on the Internet: at LWW.com. Lippincott Williams & Wilkins customer service representatives are available from 8:30 am to 6 pm, EST.

10 9 8

Preface to the Fourth Edition

The third and last edition of *The Hand: Examination and Diagnosis* was published more than 20 years ago by the American Society for Surgery of the hand. Hand surgery is a dynamic specialty. Prodigious scientific knowledge related to hand anatomy and surgery and new innovations have evolved in the last two decades. In keeping current with novel scientific developments, the American Society for Surgery of the Hand's Publication and Products Advisory Committee (PPAC), under the aegis of the Education Division, espoused the mission of updating this publication. The PPAC members whose names are listed on the previous page have been instrumental in bringing in much of the material contained within the pages of this book.

This publication is intended to unravel the beauty and mystery of complex hand anatomy for the hand surgery learner and to provide the reader with cutting edge information about common clinical hand conditions. Hence, the book is organized into two main sections: one on anatomy and another on examination and clinical conditions of the hand. The first section describes hand anatomy beginning superficially in the skin and proceeding deep to the bone, whereas the examination and clinical conditions section discusses diagnosis and treatment of injuries and diseases of these anatomical structures. The companion electronic lecture features a power point presentation about "Hand Anatomy its Relation to Injury and Disease" that is complimentary to the print publication.

We intended for this book to perpetuate the legacy of preceding editions. We revised it to be condensed yet comprehensive and classic yet current. We trust that the reader will find the encompassed material to be edifying, enlightening, and enriching. We hope that this book will be a constant companion to hand surgery students at many educational levels, in their pursuit of providing excellent quality care for their patients.

Ghazi Rayan, MD
Edward Akelman, MD

Acknowledgments

The authors thank Tara Havenga and Mark Anderson from the ASSH central office for their administrative help and strategic planning for this publication and Basil Rayan for his technical help in the production of the electronic version of this publication.

Contents

Part III: Examination and Clinical Conditions

CHAPTER **1**

The Hand and Hand Surgery

Nowhere else in the body does anatomy transform more to function than the hand. The combination of anatomy and biomechanics along with musculoskeletal, nerve, and vascular systems are all integrated into the delicate and intricate human hand.

THE HAND

Whether one looks at the classic art of Michelangelo and Leonardo da Vinci or the modern art of Picasso and Chagall, hands are depicted in various functional and expressive settings. Artists for generations have used their hands as expressive tools of their vision. From a scientific perspective, Dr. J. William Littler, one of the icons of hand surgery, has eloquently demonstrated by his own hand drawings the fine architecture and interrelationships of the many anatomic structures of the hand. The hand is a window to the body and mirror to many systemic diseases. Many organ system ailments may be evaluated and diagnosed through hand examination. Neurologic diseases manifest themselves with muscle atrophy and sensory loss. Cardiovascular diseases are diagnosed with digital cyanosis or splinter hemorrhages; pulmonary conditions may be identified by digital clubbing; and gastrointestinal nutritional disorders are demonstrated in scurvy (Vitamin C deficiency) by the presence of vascular purpura.

As with any other organ, assessment of the hand requires applying the basic principles of physical examination. Inspection, palpation, percussion, and auscultation all can and should be utilized in the complete evaluation of the hand. The art of observation may show changes in pigmentation, carcinomas of the skin, malnutrition, muscle wasting, and the consequences of trauma. Nowhere else in the musculoskeletal system can palpation of parts of the hand more readily demonstrate pathology. Virtually all structures are within the examiner's grasp. With a thorough knowledge of anatomy, the location of a patient's symptoms can direct the physician to the underlying pathology. Pain in the anatomic snuffbox is pathognomonic of a scaphoid fracture. Examining a mass may allow the physician to consider a fluid filled ganglion, a firm but pliable lipoma, or the subungual hypersensitivity of a glomus tumor. Auscultation can be used to hear the thrill of an aneurysm.

Imagine the difficulty of living or interacting in an environment without the amenities that our hands bring to our lives. Besides the obvious use of our hands for sensation and grasp, gestures are used commonly for communication. With certain hand motions one can communicate positive or negative feelings. Parents point a finger to emphasize a certain point. Hands not only have the ability to sample our environment but also to evaluate it in numerous ways. Sensibility is a complex function that encompasses fine touch, deep pressure, and the ability to perceive temperature. Our hands protect us from harmful influences through the interneuron spinal reflex arc. When we touch an exceedingly hot object the reflex causes our hands to automatically pull away. It is not until milliseconds later that we actually appreciate the perception of burning heat. As our hands perceive vibration, the spectrum is not simple touch, but a complicated system involving our central nervous system. One can feel the purr of a cat or the roar of an engine. We can exert tremendous force with a hand grasp. Conversely the fine manipulations of our fingertips allow us to type, text, and generate harmonious musical sounds. The hand of a violinist wields the bow across the cello and with complex manipulations, and coordinated efforts between both hands, generate incredible musical sounds.

HISTORY

Hand surgery can be traced back to Hippocrates (460–370 BC) who described methods for treating hand fractures and injuries. He is credited as the first to identify fractures of the distal radius and carpal dislocations. His methods of wound care still apply, in a broad sense, to this day. Though Hippocrates is given appropriate credit for his influence in the field of medicine in general, when looking back at history, he can be considered to have great influence on hand surgery. He described the classic clubbing of fingers seen in pulmonary disease. Galen's (129–200 AD) interest in anatomy, neurology, and the circulatory system provided much of the early practical hand information. Galen more accurately described hand infections and fabricated an ointment made out of wax and oil.

The science of human anatomy was refined in the 16th century by Andreas Vesalius (1513–1564), a Flemish practitioner who made detailed descriptions and illustrations of dissected human cadavers. In the 16th century, Ambroise Paré (1509–1590) further popularized and advanced the treatment of infections and open wounds. His principles of wound care and irrigation helped improving the care of many patients with severe hand infections and gangrene. The tourniquet, an instrument integral to hand surgery, was invented by the French surgeon Jean-Louis Petit. Inspecting the bloodless field of a tourniquet, Petit was able to accurately describe the anatomy associated with carpal injuries. To this day the use of a tourniquet minimizes blood loss and allows clear visualization, precise dissection, and protection of important neurovascular structures

Much to the credit of Dr. Sterling Bunnell (Fig. 1-1) from the United States, World War II provided an impetus and the necessity to establish hand surgery as a specialty by itself. As Bunnell prefaced in the second edition of his classic text *Surgery of the Hand*, major general Norman Kirk, the Surgeon General of the army, recognized the importance of saving the hands of injured soldiers. During the time of war the specialty of hand surgery began to blossom as teams of physicians, medics, and therapists began a coordinated effort to salvage injured hands that otherwise would have "remained crippled." Dr. Bunnell reported that he helped in the reconstruction of 20,000 hands of soldiers during the war. He recognized the specific details of the hand that "necessitates training and correlation of the whole

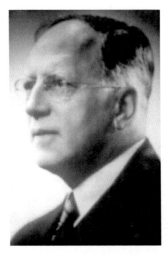

FIGURE 1-1 Sterling Bunnell, the founder of hand surgery.

problem–skin, bones, joints, nerves, tendons, mechanics, and biologics, the working unit, function as a whole and the social aspect." He went on to say that "in man, the purpose of the upper extremities is to place its most important part, the hand where it can work."

The American Society for Surgery of the Hand was founded in 1946 by a group of surgeons, lead by Bunnell, who had devoted a great part of their lives to helping patients with hand injuries. With varied backgrounds and different types of training, these seminal hand surgeons realized that the complexities of the hand required, and would benefit from, an organization dedicated to the study, research, and advancement of hand disorders.

THE HAND SURGEON

A hand surgeon requires training and certification well beyond that of the primary board certification. To be recognized as a member of the American Society for Surgery of the Hand, each surgeon must complete an accredited residency in orthopedic surgery, plastic surgery, or general surgery and should complete an additional year of training in an accredited Hand fellowship program.

The attestation does not end there; the hand surgeon must pass an examination of "The Certificate of Added Qualifications in Surgery of the Hand" and demonstrate a dedication to the specialty by proving an interest and a specialization in disorders of the upper extremity. The hand surgeon can treat upper extremity disorders of patients of all ages from the newborn to the elderly. The hand surgeon provides emergent care for amputations, fractures, and ligament, tendon, nerve, and arterial injuries. The hand surgeon can reconstruct upper extremity birth defects, arthritic diseases, and paralytic hands. A hand surgeon must understand the interrelationship between all the tissues from the fingertip to the shoulder.

The advent of microsurgery in the 1960s allowed the hand surgeon to address injuries of intricate structures and helped reconstruct the mangled and severely injured limbs. Microsurgery is a term applied to the use of a microscope in the operating room that allows the surgeon to visualize the small nerves and arteries that provide sensation and blood supply to the digits and hand. Drs Harold Kleinert and Harry Buncke popularized the techniques of microsurgery in the United States. The former reported the first revascularization of a partial amputation in 1963 and the latter, using animal models, helped develop the techniques and instrumentation for replantation. Since that time, not only have severed digits, hands, and arms been replanted, but microsurgery allowed the proliferation of free tissue transfers. Muscle, bone, and skin can now be moved from one area of the body to another for covering defects. The use of free tissue transfer or free flaps has now been expanded to allograft (from one person to another) hand transplantation.

The varied backgrounds from which hand surgeons originate parallels the varied pathology that hand surgeons treat. Hand surgeons utilizing orthopedic surgery background can address fractures and dislocations; hand surgeons utilizing plastic surgery background may perform soft tissue repair, skin tumor resection, and flap coverage; hand surgeons utilizing neurosurgery background can repair and reconstruct peripheral nerves; and hand surgeons utilizing vascular surgery background can repair vessels as small as 0.5 mm in diameter. The hand surgeon addresses all these injuries when replanting a severed digit or limb. A hand surgeon therefore needs to be adept at treating not only the skeletal system but also skin, tendons, nerves, and vessels.

Hand surgery has an international background and the specialty has been advanced from contributions worldwide. European surgeons have developed advanced techniques for fracture fixation. Surgeons from South America have popularized vascularized bone grafts to treat nonunion and avascular necrosis. Hand surgeons from Asia and the Pacific Rim have advanced our treatment of brachial plexus and neuromuscular lesions. The worldwide network has proliferated across the globe with the attendance of combined and international meetings.

To address conditions of the hand, the physician requires understanding and ability to treat disorders of the hand, wrist, forearm, and for some practitioners the elbow and shoulder. The interrelationship of each component of the upper extremity is integral for diagnosing and treating its disorders. Though the specialty is termed hand surgery the vast majority of disorders and injuries of the hand can be treated without surgery. The hand surgeon rarely works in a vacuum and often interacts with other specialists, including radiologists, neurologists, rheumatologists, and certified hand therapists who are concerned with hand rehabilitation. Medications, exercise, and splints can enrich the care and cure of many disorders. Surgery is relegated to those conditions that do not respond to conservative measures or in situations where injuries are severe and surgical intervention will help facilitate an earlier return to function and activities of daily living

The complexities of our hands have inspired the birth and the growth of an entire specialty within medicine, namely hand surgery. The coordination of multiple elements that allow our hands to function and communicate requires the skills of hand specialists who can meet that challenge.

CHAPTER **2**

Functional Anatomy and Biomechanics

A concise knowledge of hand and forearm anatomy is essential to competently perform an examination of this region. The arm and forearm position the hand to allow for the performance of the essential activities of daily living. In addition to these dexterous motor activities, the hand serves as a major sensory organ to explore the environment and convey information to the brain. These actions are possible because of the hand's unique anatomy and functional design.

FUNCTIONAL UNITS

The hand can be divided into three digital functional units: the thumb, index and long fingers, and ring and small fingers. Most fine motor actions are performed by the first and third units, the thumb and index and/or long finger(s) with the small and ring finger serving as a base for performance of this action by these digits.

The independence of the thumb ray is made possible by its position on the hand, its bony structure, and independent musculature. The lateral position and orientation of the thumb at rest is in an anatomical plane separate from the fingers, which allows the key motion of opposition. The ability of the thumb to assume and work from this position is directly related to its underlying boney architecture. The bones of this digit are markedly different than

| TABLE 2-1 | Muscles of the Thumb |

Intrinsic	Extrinsic
Adductor pollicis	Abductor pollicis longus
First dorsal interosseous	Extensor pollicis brevis
Flexor pollicis brevis	Extensor pollicis longus
Abductor pollicis brevis	Flexor pollicis longus
Opponens pollicis	

the four fingers, with the scaphoid, trapezium, and metacarpal allowing for a mobile base by unique joint geometry. This geometry is particularly evident in the double opposing saddle configuration of the joint between the thumb metacarpal base and the trapezium, which allows for flexion–extension, abduction–adduction, rotation, and circumduction. The flexor pollicis longus muscle, unlike other digital flexors, originates independently low in the forearm and because of its vector of force participates in not only flexion but also pronation. In addition to this independent muscle the thumb is motored by three additional extrinsic muscles and five intrinsic muscles (Table 2-1).

Opposition, noted above as a key motion of the thumb unit, is a term that requires definition. In positional astronomy this term describes the phenomenon of two celestial bodies being on opposite sides of the sky when viewed from a set point. In hand surgery this term describes the change in position of the thumb, together with its metacarpal. During this change the thumb moves from its position of rest, lateral to the index finger, to a new position in front of the fingers by a combination of rotation, abduction, and varying degrees of flexion. At rest or in adduction the nail plate of the thumb is directed laterally or dorsally, in full opposition the nail plate rotates anterior so the pulp of the thumb faces the pulp of the fingers (Fig. 2-1). A practical test of the integrity of this function is to direct the patient to pick up a grape-size ball between the long finger and the thumb pulps (Fig. 2-2).

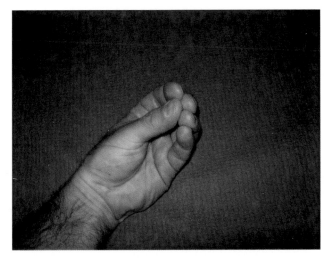

FIGURE 2-1 Hand demonstrating the combined motion of thumb rotation, abduction, and variable flexion required to accomplish opposition.

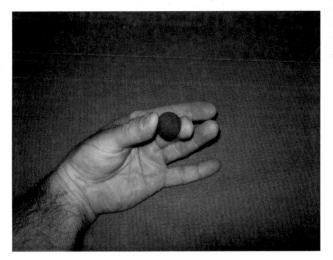

FIGURE 2-2 Simple maneuver which may be used to test for opposition.

The second functional unit consists of the index and long fingers that are often used in concert with the thumb to perform fine motor motions. Of these two digits the index finger is designed and positioned more independently than the long finger and exhibits more rotation at its metacarpophalangeal joint than the other three fingers. The independence of the index finger is facilitated by the separation of the muscle bellies of the flexor digitorum profundus and superficialis of this digit from those of other fingers. In addition to these extrinsic muscles, the index finger is motored by the largest interosseous muscle, the first dorsal interosseous. This muscle originates on the ulnar border of the thumb metacarpal and inserts on the palmar plate of the metacarpophalangeal joint, the lateral tubercle of the base of the proximal phalanx of the index finger and the extensor hood. This muscle has both deep and superficial heads with the deep head causing mainly flexion pinch between the thumb and the index finger, and the superficial head providing abduction. Within the complex physiology of the various types of opposition of thumb and index, the dorsal interosseous muscle acts as a stabilizer.

The third and final functional unit of the hand is the ring and small fingers. This unit grants the strong motor action required during powerful grasp. As previously noted these two digits also act together to form a stable platform for fine motor tasks performed by the other two functional units acting in concert. This activity is facilitated by the mobility observed at the fourth and fifth carpometacarpal (CMC) joints that allow palmar cupping as the fingers are being flexed. This motion is enhanced by the activity of the oblique opponens digiti minimi muscle that acts on the fifth CMC joint and is the only muscle that acts on the CMC joints alone. This muscle is optimally positioned to flex and rotate the fifth metacarpal bone about its long axis thereby enhancing the natural arch observed in the metacarpals.

ARCHES OF THE HAND

Architecturally there are three important arches of the hand: the longitudinal arch, the proximal transverse arch, and the distal transverse arch (Fig. 2-3). It is important to understand that these arches exist not only because of bony structure but also because of the influence of the multiple soft tissue motors that drive hand function. In essence many of the functions of the hand are

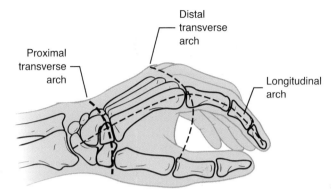

FIGURE 2-3 Schematic drawing that depicts the three arches of the hand: the longitudinal arch, proximal transverse arch, and distal transverse arch.

completed by alterations to the varying degrees of these arches. Because the arches represent the symbiosis of both bony and soft tissue structures they may be disrupted by both direct trauma and by distant nerve injury. Restoration of disrupted arches may require soft tissue and bony stabilization or reconstruction.

For each ray of the four fingers the longitudinal arch spans from the fixed CMC articulation to the mobile digits, with the MP articulation acting as the keystone; the MP joint is therefore essential for support of the longitudinal arch. The longitudinal arch is best observed by following the middle finger ray, which along with its metacarpal forms the anatomical axis of the hand. This digit appears to deepen with finger flexion and flatten with finger extension as the more mobile rays move to each side of the axis.

The proximal transverse arch is at the level of the CMC joint of the axial middle finger metacarpal with the keystone being the capitate. This arch is relatively immobile and remains domed even when the hand is maximally opened.

The distal transverse arch is formed by the metacarpal heads of the four fingers which are bound together by the inter palmar plate ligament connecting the palmar plates of each MP articulation. This arch is mobile with the first, fourth, and fifth metacarpals rotating around the relatively fixed heads of both the second (index) and third (middle) metacarpals to either flatten or increase the arc or the arch. In full finger extension, the arch is flattened with finger flexion the arch is maximized.

The arches both support and participate in the complex movements of the functional units of the hand which allow it to perform so many tasks we take for granted.

MOVEMENTS OF THE HAND

The hand is capable of many movements as well as variation in strength and precision. These movements are intimately related to the complex anatomy which exists in this relatively confined space, coupled with precise sensory input. These movements have been scientifically evaluated and studied from various points of view. The digital movement along the longitudinal arch has been postulated to be guided by the interrelationship of three mathematical elements: the Fibonacci sequence, the golden ratio, and the equiangular spiral.

The thumb is capable of flexion at its MP and IP joints as well as the base of the metacarpal at its articulation with the trapezium. Radial abduction and adduction of the thumb occurs from and to the index metacarpal via the articulation of the base of the metacarpal and the trapezium, the trapeziometacarpal joint. Extension may take place in the thumb at the IP joint, the MCP joint, and the trapeziometacarpal joint. In addition the thumb, as previously described, can perform the complex motion of opposition.

Each finger is capable of flexion and extension at the distal interphalangeal (DIP) joint, proximal interphalangeal (PIP) joint, and at the MP joint. The MP joint is also capable of abduction and adduction, as well as circumduction. The capability for circumduction is most developed in the index finger. Since the long finger ray forms the axis of the hand, motion of the other fingers toward this digit in the coronal plane, that is, frontal plane, is termed adduction while movement away is termed abduction.

Functional movement of the digits of the hand cannot be considered independent of wrist motion. Maximal extension of the fingers is associated with slight flexion of the wrist, whereas flexion of the fingers as maximally expressed in the formation of a fist is associated with the extension of the wrist. In addition the wrist may perform radial and ulnar deviation in the frontal plane and

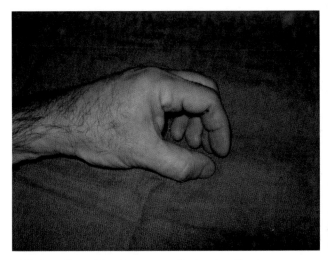

FIGURE 2-4 The position of rest assumed by the relaxed hand.

circumduction where the moving wrist forms the apex of a cone and the tip of the long finger describes the circumference.

The inactive hand normally assumes the position of rest. In this position the hand is slightly extended and ulnarly deviated at the wrist, and the fingers are flexed at the DIP, PIP, and MP joints (Fig. 2-4). The thumb assumes slight abduction and the pulp comes into proximity or touches the radial aspect of the PIP joint of the index finger.

In contrast, in the position of function the hand is poised for rapid movement to various positions of activity. The wrist is more extended, the MP joints are extended and abducted, and the interphalangeal joints are slightly flexed (Fig. 2-5). The thumb is strongly abducted, slightly extended at the MP joint, slightly flexed at the IP joint, and the thumb metacarpal is rotated so that its radio-ulnar plane is perpendicular to the radio-ulnar plane of the finger metacarpals. This position is the safe position for splinting of the hand after injury and many surgical procedures.

More grossly, the movements of the hand can be consolidated into non-prehensile or prehensile. Non-prehensile movements

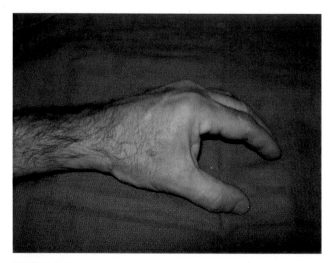

FIGURE 2-5 The safe position.

consist of pushing or pulling an object without the use of grip. In contrast, prehension would involve grasping, carrying, and releasing an object. Precise manipulative acts of prehension usually involve the thumb while prehensile movements that exclude the thumb usually consist of some form of power grip/grasp.

There are three distinct types of non-manipulative prehensile power grips. In the first or hook grip, the fingers bring the object against the palm and the object is held with the hand in line with the forearm. The fingers are flexed at the PIP and DIP joints while the MP joints are in neutral position; the wrist is in slight ulnar deviation and extention. The thumb is essentially non-functional in this type of grip which is utilized to carry objects such as a suitcase. Primary muscles involved in this type of grip are the flexor digitorum superficialis and profundus, extensor pollicis longus and brevis, extensor digitorum comminus, fourth lumbrical, and the interossei.

In the other three prehensile non-manipulative grips (cylindrical and spherical grasp, and fist grip), the fingers are used to hold an object in the palm of the hand. The palm contours to the object by movement of the mobile distal transverse arch and the thumb provides an additional surface to control the object by adducting against it. Cylindrical grasp is the type of grip used to hold a can of soda. In this grasp the thumb is held in opposition and the fingers are adducted and flexed at the interphalangeal joints. The intrinsic thenar muscles, flexor pollicis longus, adductor pollicis, and flexor digitorum profundus, are active during this type of grasp. Spherical grasp is used to hold round objects, and in this grasp the thumb is again held in opposition but the fingers assume a flexed and abducted position. Because the same muscles are active in spherical grasp as cylindrical grasp, some investigators do not distinguish between these two forms of grasp.

The final form of prehensile non-manipulative grip is the fist grip. This is the type of grip utilized to hold a narrow object into the palm of the hand such as a broom handle. In this grip the thumb is again in opposition, but the fingers are flexed at the MP joints in addition to the interphalangeal joints.

Prehensile manipulative pinch patterns include key, chuck, closed round pinch, and closed elongated pinch (Fig. 2-6A–D). Key or lateral pinch is used when a thin object is held between the palmar surface of the thumb and the lateral side of the index proximal phalanx and/or metacarpal. This form of pinch is an imprecise manipulative pinch that importantly can be attained by tenodesis to achieve surgically some function following spinal cord injury. Chuck pinch is also a less precise form of pinch where the distal pulp of the opposed thumb meets the distal pulps of the index and middle fingers when they are in continuity. The closed round pinch is a precise pinch that permits picking up small objects between the index or long finger and the thumb. In this pinch the thumb metacarpal rotates, carrying with it the proximal and distal phalanges of the thumb, which are held in slight flexion so that its pulp touches that of the index or long finger. During this pinch the index finger flexes at MP and interphalangeal joints and the wrist assume a position of moderate extension. The closed elongated pinch is a modification of the closed round pinch where the distal phalanges of the thumb and index or long finger are held in extension instead of flexion as their pulps converge together. These final two forms of pinch are used to pick up small objects or perform precise maneuvers such as threading a needle.

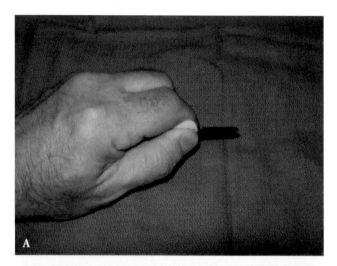

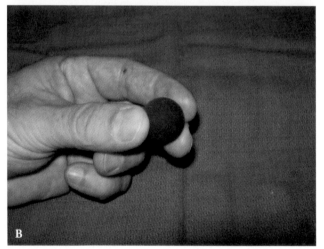

FIGURE 2-6 The four types of pinch the intact hand can perform: **A:** key Pinch, **B:** Chuck pinch (*continued*)

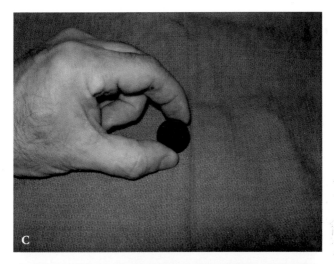

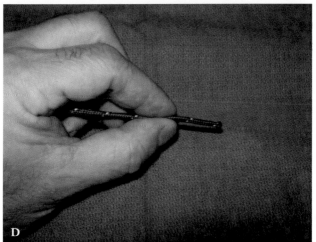

FIGURE 2-6 (*Continued*) **C:** closed round pinch, and **D:** closed elongated pinch. (All photographs are courtesy of Steve Peterson MD).

SURGICAL IMPLICATONS

Anatomical restoration is necessary for functional recovery. Consequently the basis of hand surgery is founded in a complete knowledge of the anatomy of the hand and how it relates to function. Surgical approaches in the hand should be targeted so as to minimize trauma to adjacent structures and minimize postoperative scar and edema that could restrict motion or delay therapy. Appreciation of the interactions between soft tissues and bone is required as well as the ability to treat each of the multiple tissue types present in the hand. This brief introduction to the functional anatomy of the hand will hopefully serve as basis for future more in-depth exploration of this complex topic.

CHAPTER 3

Perionychium

The perionychium encompasses the nail plate and the surrounding soft tissues. This fingernail component includes specialized skin structures around the nail plate, as well as the cellular structures responsible for nail growth and maintenance. The nail unit or perionychium is important for tactile touch, regulation of peripheral circulation, and protection of the finger tip. The hard nail plate facilitates compression of the pulp or finger pad between what is being touched and the nail plate, enhancing the network of pulp sensory nerve endings to evaluate the object of touch. Because of its location at the tip of the finger, the perionychium is vulnerable and is the most frequently injured part of the hand.

The perionychium is made up of the following structures (Fig. 3-1).

NAIL PLATE
This hard structure is composed of onchyn, a keratinous material that is left after the death of germinal matrix cells which then form the growing nail. The nail plate is resistant to weak acids and bases and forms a protective cover over the nail bed.

NAIL BED
The nail bed is the soft tissue deep to the nail plate and consists of the germinal matrix and the sterile matrix. The germinal matrix is a group of cells that produce 90% of the overlying nail by the process of cell death and transference of cells superficially to form the nail plate. This unique structure comprises the proximal portion of the nail bed, and its distal extent is the lunula, which is

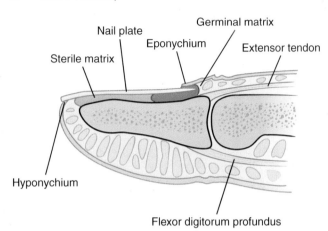

FIGURE 3-1 Anatomy of the perionychium.

the white moon-shaped structure seen at the base of the nail. The germinal matrix's deepest layer of cells rests directly on the periosteum of the distal phalanx; hence fractures of the distal phalanx can damage this matrix and disrupt nail growth.

The sterile matrix is located in the distal portion of the nail bed and produces a thin layer of cells that contribute to the formation of the deep surface of the nail plate and increases its adherence to the nail bed. Injuries to the sterile matrix can cause nail bed deformities such as ridging.

NAIL FOLD

The nail fold or socket is a strong structure that hosts the proximal portion of the nail plate and contributes to its stability. It is made up of the dorsal roof, which is the end portion of the eponychium, and the ventral floor, which is the germinal matrix of the nail bed.

EPONYCHIUM

The eponychium is the specialized soft tissue located proximal to the nail plate. It includes the dorsal half of the nail fold, into which the hard nail plate is inserted. The thin filmy extension of the eponychium onto the nail plate is called the nail vest or cuticle.

PARONYCHIUM

The paronychium is the skin on either side of the nail at its lateral and medial edges. It may provide some stability to the nail plate.

HYPONYCHIUM

The hyponychium at the finger tip is the area where the finger pulp meets the sterile matrix at its distal edge. This keratinous area of skin contains a high concentration of nerves, vessels, lymphocytes, and polymorphonuclear cells. The latter cells are thought to protect this vulnerable area against infection.

BLOOD AND NERVE SUPPLY OF THE PERIONYCHIUM

The nerve supply to the fingertip is from dorsal and volar branches of the digital nerves, which travel on the volar (radial and ulnar) aspect of the finger. At the base of the nail, these arborize, sending both dorsal and volar branches to form a network of sensitive nerve endings. Additionally, the fingertip contains unique neurovascular apparatus consisting of glomus bodies, which are intertwined objects of tiny nerves and blood vessels that control blood flow at the perionychium. Glomus bodies are located both within the nail bed, where they function as temperature regulators, and throughout the fingertip.

The digital arteries of the finger, which course on the volar side of the finger, similarly branch just proximal to the nail base toward the dorsal and the volar sides of the finger. Capillaries in the pulp form end loops to provide a richly vascular network for the finger tip.

CHAPTER 4

Skin

The skin, or integument, is the largest human organ representing in the average adult 8% of the total body mass. It is a highly specialized organ that serves as an interface between the body and its environment. The skin is essential for life, and changes in its appearance reflect not only responses to external influences but also mirror internal systemic disease.

HISTOLOGY

Microscopically, skin is formed by two intimate but distinct tissues: keratinized stratified squamous epithelium, the epidermis, and a deeper layer of moderately dense connective tissue, the dermis. The thickness of both the epidermis and dermis varies in different anatomical areas of the body. Variation in epidermal thickness is grossly obvious when comparing the palm, where the epidermis can be as thick as 1.5 mm with the dorsum of the hand where it may be as thin as 0.1 mm. This combination of epidermis and dermis serves as an effective barrier against microbial invasion and dehydration, as well as physical assault. Skin also contains and is penetrated by adnexal structures such as nails, sweat glands, sebaceous glands, and hair follicles (Fig. 4-1) and is heavily populated by a variety of sensory end organs.

Normal hormonal changes may affect the appearance and function of specific areas of the skin, as can the age, state of health, sun exposure, and various other aspects of an individual's life. In addition to normal changes these exposures can also play a role in the development of certain skin disease states.

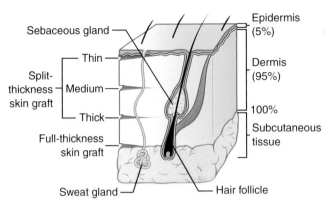

FIGURE 4-1 Schematic drawing demonstrating the relationships of epidermis, dermis, and adnexal structures in glabrous skin.

GROSS ANATOMY

The skin covering the hand is adaptively different from the skin in other parts of the body. On the dorsum of the hand the skin contains hair follicles (hirsute skin) and is held in place by a loose layer of areolar tissue, allowing more mobility than the palmar skin. Dorsally there are areas of redundancy over the joints which tend to wrinkle when the hand is extended and stretch with flexion. Numerous large veins traverse within the loose areolar tissue of the dorsum of the hand. Relative to the volar surface of the hand the dorsum is sparsely populated with sensory nerve endings.

On the volar surface of the hand the skin is thickened, devoid of hair (glabrous skin), and shows characteristic whorls, or fingerprints, and flexion creases. The dermis on the palm, unlike that on the dorsum, is connected with multiple minute vertical fibrous bands to the underlying palmar fascial complex resulting in a relatively immobile surface that greatly facilitates grip and allows manipulation of small objects.

There are two transverse creases on the palm that correspond to the underlying metacarpophalangeal joints (Fig. 4-2). The most

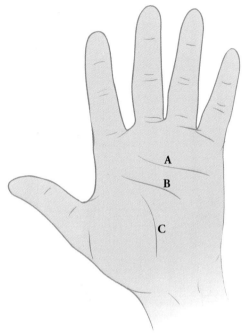

FIGURE 4-2 Line drawing demonstrating the major three palmar creases and their relationship to the underlying bones and articulations. **A:** Distal palmar crease. **B:** Proximal palmar crease. **C:** Thenar crease.

distal transverse palmar crease overlies the metacarpophalangeal joints of the ring and small fingers, while the proximal transverse crease lies at the level of the metacarpophalangeal joints of the index and long fingers. A third crease, the palmar thenar crease, extends from the first web space to the wrist crease and corresponds to the basal joints of the thumb and is associated with the complex motion of opposition.

A single palmar crease is present in approximately 3% of the population with twice incidence in males versus females. While a single palmar crease is often a normal finding it may also be associated with a variety of syndromes, including Downs, Aarskog, Cohen, Fetal Alcohol, Rubella, Turner, Klinefelter, Trisomy 13, and Cri du chat, as well as pseudohypoparathyroidism and gonadal dysgenesis.

In addition to the three primary palmar creases there are also creases anatomically located over the four fingers opposite the middle of the proximal phalanges, the palmar digital creases. These creases are associated with deeper fascial structures that anchor the distal palm and finger webs. In contrast to the fingers, the palmar digital crease of the abducted thumb is longitudinally oriented and is slightly proximal to the underlying metacarpophalangeal joint. Further distally is the interphalangeal joint crease of the thumb, and the proximal interphalangeal joint and distal interphalangeal joint creases of the fingers. These creases are directly over their corresponding joints and serve as useful surgical landmarks. The proximal interphalangeal creases and interphalangeal joint crease of the thumb are usually evident as two distinct creases in contrast to the palmar digital and distal interphalangeal creases which are usually single.

Supernumerary digital creases have been reported in less than 1% of the general population. The presence of extra and missing digital creases in patients with normal joint anatomy indicates that genetic factors contribute to digital crease formation. Specific genetic changes that have been associated with supernumerary crease formation are partial deletions of chromosome 1q, partial trisomy of 13q, cerebro-oculo-facial syndrome, sickle cell disease, and Alagille syndrome, where up to one-third of individuals with this syndrome may present with supernumerary creases.

Another notable feature of the hand is the four web spaces that are present between the five digits of the hand which are numerically numbered from 1 to 4 from radial to ulnar. These spaces consist of thin glabrous skin dorsally and thick glabrous skin palmary. The distal extents of the three webs associated with the four fingers are in continuity with the palmar digital creases of the adjacent fingers. In contrast the first web space between the thumb and the index finger does not associate with the palmar digital crease of the index finger but instead extends from the palmar digital crease of the thumb to the proximal palmar crease.

Whorls or papillary ridges are confined in the hand to the palm and flexor surfaces of the digits where they form parallel and curved arrays separated by narrow furrows. Along the midline of each ridge the apertures of sweat glands, which are most dense in the palm and finger tips of the hand, open at regular intervals. Each visible ridge corresponds microscopically to an underlying pattern of dermal papillae which anchor the epidermis and dermis together.

These individually distinct patterns of ridges and furrows are formed early during fetal development and in the absence of trauma or certain disease states are stable throughout life allowing for their use in identification as fingerprints. That fingerprint patterns are not entirely a genetic characteristic is evidenced by the individuality of patterns even in monozygotic twins. Other factors that seem to play a role in finger development during limb development include nutrition, parental blood pressure, fetal position in the womb, and the growth rate of the fingers at the end of the first trimester. The clarity of these distinctive whorls after birth may also be affected by a variety of conditions including eczema, leprosy, hypohidrotic ectodermal dysplasia, adult acanthosis nigricans, celiac disease, scleroderma, and Darier disease.

CHAPTER 5

Subcutaneous Tissue

The superficial fascia is also known as the subdermis or hypodermis. It is the layer of tissue directly beneath the dermis. Histologically, it has fat cells, fibroblasts, and macrophages. It is comprised of connective and adipose tissues. It may contain neurovascular structures in varying proportions depending on the location in the body or hand. The subcutaneous tissue in most of the body acts as a reservoir for the storage of fat and provides insulation. In the hand, the subcutaneous tissue is more specialized and its function varies depending on its location whether dorsal or palmar.

The dorsal subcutaneous tissue of the hand is located in a narrow space between the skin and the deep fascia that consists mostly of loose areolar connective tissue and some adipose tissue (Fig. 5-1). It is loosely attached to the dermis, a characteristic that is responsible for a great deal of mobility of the dorsal skin. The subcutaneous space of the dorsum of the hand contains blood vessels, mostly veins of the superficial venous system and the companion lymphatic system.

Palmar subcutaneous tissue of the hand is located in a very thick space that consists mostly of adipose tissue coalesced as lobules of fat separated by fibrous tissue septa (Fig. 5-2). It contains numerous, small, minute but strong fibrous bands (Grapaw fibers) that span the depth of the space and connect the dermis to the underlying structures, including the fibrous tendon sheath and periosteum. This arrangement contributes to the stability of the palmar skin during pinch and grasp.

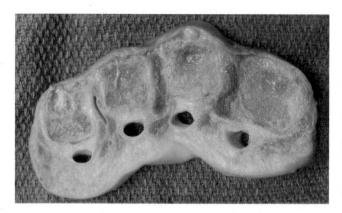

FIGURE 5-1 Cross-sectional anatomy of the hand at the distal palmar level showing the dorsal narrow subcutaneous space and thick palmar subcutaneous space.(Pictures are courtesy of Ghazi Rayan MD.)

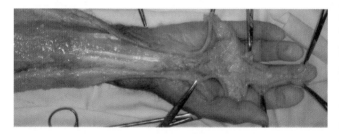

FIGURE 5-2 Palmar subcutaneous thick space of the forearm, hand, and digit showing the abundance of adipose tissue that is coalesced as lobules of fat separated by fibrous tissue septa.

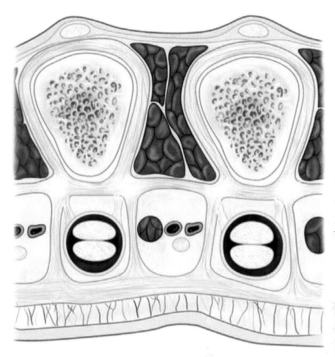

FIGURE 5-3 Illustration of the cross-sectional anatomy of the hand showing the difference between the thin dorsal versus thick palmar subcutaneous spaces.

CHAPTER **6**

Deep Fascia

DORSAL ASPECT

The deep fascia of the dorsal aspect of the hand constitutes a layer of retinacular tissue or dorsal aponeurosis that incorporates and binds the extensor tendons of the digits. It contains the juncturae tendinea that connects the digital extensor tendons. This layer separates the dorsal subcutaneous space from the dorsal subaponeurotic space. The dorsal subcutaneous space contains sensory cutaneous nerves along with the venous and lymphatic systems. The dorsal subaponeurotic space contains the dorsal digital arteries. The floor of the dorsal subaponeurotic space is made up of the interosseous muscles and metacarpal bones.

PALMAR ASPECT

The deep fascia of the palmar aspect of the hand, known as the palmar fascial complex (Fig. 6-1), is made up of radial, ulnar, and central aponeuroses, palmodigital fascia, and digital fascia. While the palmar fascial complex can be divided into defined structures, it is important to remember that it is a continuous fibrous skeleton.

- The central aponeurosis is triangular shaped (Fig. 6-2), with the apex at the wrist level and serves as the insertion of the palmaris longus (when it is present). It is composed of longitudinal, transverse, and vertical fibers.
  - The longitudinal fibers (Fig. 6-3) make up the pretendinous bands that course superficial and parallel to the deeper flexor tendons. These bands extend from the wrist level to the base of each digit. There are three of these longitudinal bands within the central aponeurosis, one for each index, middle, and ring fingers. Distally, each band bifurcates at the level of

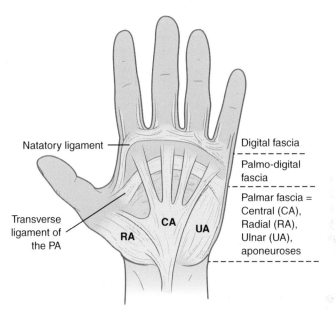

FIGURE 6-1 Main components of the palmar fascial complex.

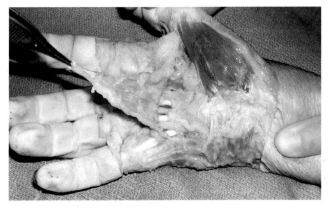

FIGURE 6-2 The central aponeurosis reflected from its proximal attachment. (Picture courtesy of Ghazi Rayan MD).

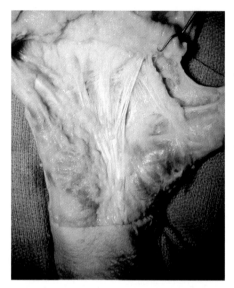

FIGURE 6-3 The three pretendinous bands of the central aponeurosis. (Picture courtesy of Ghazi Rayan MD).

the metacarpophalangeal joint, and each split portion of the longitudinal band divides into three layers. The most superficial layer inserts into the skin of the distal palm. The second layer continues distally towards the digit as the spiral band. These fibers rotate 90 degrees as they pass into the finger. The third layer inserts dorsally at the metacarpophalangeal joints.

- The transverse fibers make up the transverse ligament of the palmar aponeurosis (TLPA) that runs dorsal and perpendicular to the pretendinous bands from the ulnar side of the small finger to the radial side of the index finger. The distal transverse fibers are the natatory ligament (Fig. 6-4), which is located at the palmodigital creases.
- There are two types of vertical fibers: multiple small bands and larger septa. The multiple small bands are located in the subcutaneous space and connect the palmar fascial complex to the dermis. The larger vertical fibers are known as septa, of Legueu and Juvara. There are eight vertical septa, of Legueu and Juvara (Fig. 6-5), that form seven longitudinal canals: four flexor

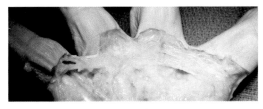

FIGURE 6-4 The natatory ligament. (Picture courtesy of Ghazi Rayan MD).

tendon and three web space canals containing the lumbrical muscles and the common digital arteries and nerves.

- The radial aponeurosis consists of the fascia overlying the thenar muscles, the thumb pretendinous band, the distal commissural ligament, and the proximal commissural ligament. The proximal commissural ligament is a continuation of the TLPA. The distal commissural ligament is the radial continuation of the natatory ligament.
- The ulnar aponeurosis consists of the fascia overlying the hypothenar muscles, the small finger pretendinous band, and the abductor digiti minimi muscle confluence distally and pisiform ligament complex proximally.
- The palmodigital fascia is the connection between the palmar and digital fascia. The most important component of this area is the middle layer of the split pretendinous band which continues as the spiral bands into the fingers. As these fibers course distally they spiral around the neurovascular bundle. The spiral bands travel first superficial then lateral and finally dorsal to the neurovascular

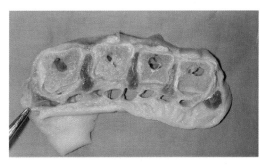

FIGURE 6-5 The septa of Legueu and Juvara. (Picture courtesy of Ghazi Rayan MD).

NORMAL

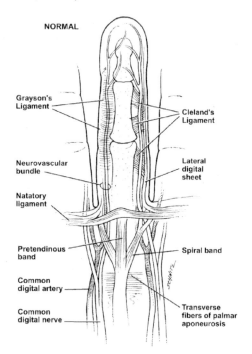

Grayson's Ligament

Cleland's Ligament

Neurovascular bundle

Lateral digital sheet

Natatory ligament

Pretendinous band

Spiral band

Common digital artery

Common digital nerve

Transverse fibers of palmar aponeurosis

FIGURE 6-6 Normal finger anatomy of fascial structures. (Reproduced from Hughes TB, Mechrefe A, Littler JW, et al. Dupuytren's disease. *J American Society Surg Hand.* 2003)

bundle and natatory ligament to continue as the lateral digital sheet of Gossett.
- The digital fascia is made up of the lateral digital sheet, Grayson ligament, and Cleland ligament (Fig. 6-6).
  - The lateral digital sheet is formed by a blending of the spiral band and fibers passing distally from the natatory ligament.
  - Grayson ligaments pass from the volar aspect of the flexor tendon sheath, palmar to the digital neurovascular bundle, to insert on the skin. To fully expose the neurovascular bundle, these ligaments should be divided.
  - Cleland ligaments pass dorsal to the digital neurovascular bundle. Together with Grayson ligaments, they anchor the skin to the digit.

7

Hand Spaces

The hand is partitioned into multiple spaces by many fascial and bony boundaries. Although seemingly complex, these hand spaces house important and separate structures from each other. Understanding the anatomy of these hand spaces is important for treating related clinical problems such as trauma, infections, inflammatory arthritic conditions, and compartment syndromes.

The various spaces of the hand include the carpal canal, digital flexor sheaths, radial and ulnar bursae, midpalmar and thenar spaces, web spaces, and dorsally the subcutaneous and subaponeurotic spaces.

CARPAL TUNNEL

The carpal canal (Fig. 7-1A–B) is the space through which the digital and thumb flexor tendons and the median nerve leave the forearm and enter the hand. A total of nine tendons (two for each finger and one for the thumb) and their tenosynovium traverse through the carpal canal. The carpal canal is quadrangular oval shaped and bordered by the carpal bones and base of 4 metacarpals dorsally, the scaphoid and trapezium radially, the hook of the hamate ulnarly, and the transverse carpal ligament volarly. The carpal tunnel is a narrow space, and when the canal contents expand the median nerve becomes compressed and ischemic, a condition known as carpal tunnel syndrome.

FLEXOR SHEATHS

Each of the digital flexor tendons is enveloped by a double-walled synovial membrane called the tendon sheath. The flexor sheath for each of the index, middle, and ring fingers extends from the distal

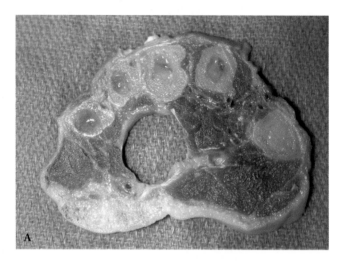

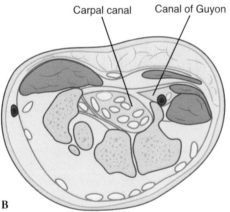

FIGURE 7-1 Anatomical cross-sectional specimen of the carpal tunnel space near its distal end **(A)** and an illustration of the tunnel further proximal **(B)**. (Picture 1A is courtesy of Ghazi Rayan MD).

palm over the MCP joint to the FDP tendon insertion into the distal phalanx. Those for the thumb and small finger extend proximally into the forearm as the radial and ulnar bursae (Fig. 7-2). The outer layer of the tendon sheath is called the parietal synovium and is

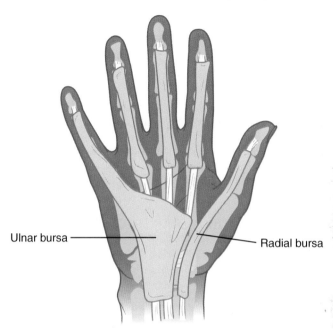

FIGURE 7-2 An illustration of the flexor tendon sheaths and ulnar and radial bursae.

surrounded by fibrous thickenings, which are termed the annular and cruciate pulleys. These pulleys provide mechanical advantage to the digit. The pulleys prevent bowstringing of the flexor tendons during finger flexion, allowing the forearm muscles to transform a relatively small amount of tendon excursion into powerful torque at the joints necessary for gripping and pinching. The inner or visceral layer of the tendon sheath is termed the epitenon and is rich with blood vessels, tendon cells (tenocytes), and collagen. This layer is closely adherent to the flexor tendon and is important for tendon gliding, nutrition, and healing.

HAND BURSAE
Radial Bursa
The FPL tendon is enveloped proximally by a thickened synovial sheath called the radial bursa. This bursa is an extension of the

thumb tendon sheath and traverses the wrist into the distal forearm. Thumb flexor tendon sheath infections, known as septic flexor tenosynovitis, therefore, can track into this bursa toward the forearm.

Ulnar Bursa

The synovial sheath surrounding the small finger flexor tendons extends into the palm, wrist, and forearm as the ulnar bursa. In some instances the small finger tendon sheath does not unite with the ulnar bursa. Occasionally, the ulnar and radial bursae are connected with one another. Because of this connection, infection in one of these bursae may reach the other, rarely forming a "horseshoe abscess."

MID PALMAR AND THENAR SPACES

These are not true or well-defined anatomic spaces but rather potential spaces that are without any synovial lining. They become more defined in cases of deep palmar infections of the hand when they are distended with purulent fluid. The midpalmar space (Fig. 7-3) is located deep to the flexor tendons and superficial to the metacarpals and interossei muscles in the mid-palm. This space is deep to the digital flexor tendons, lumbrical muscles, and common digital neurovascular bundles. The thenar space (Fig. 7-3) is another

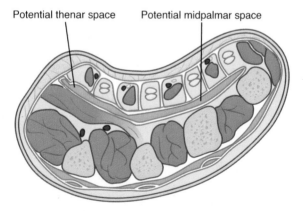

Potential thenar space   Potential midpalmar space

FIGURE 7-3 An illustration of the thenar and deep palmar spaces on the hand.

potential space that is adjacent to the mid-palmar space on one side and the thenar and adductor pollicis muscles on the other. It may communicate with the first web space. The clinical relevance of these spaces is that their knowledge helps understanding the appropriate way to treat hand infections and tumors, which may expand and violate these spaces.

PULP SPACE

The pulp space also is not true and well-defined cavity, but rather multiple adipose compartments. The subcutaneous fat that constitutes the tips of the fingers is loculated by numerous vertical bands, which create multiple closed spaces. These fibrous bands restrict the amount of swelling of the fingertip and are important clinically when excessive bleeding occurs in this location and when an infection is located in the pulp of the fingertip.

DORSAL SPACES

There are two dorsal spaces in the hand; the dorsal subcutaneous space, which is located between the extensor tendons and dermis over the dorsum of the hand and the subaponeurotic space which, is situated deep to the extensor tendons over the dorsal aspect of the finger metacarpals.

CHAPTER 8

Vascular System

The hand is supplied by two arteries: the radial and ulnar which terminate into the common digital and digital arteries (Fig. 8-1). Both arteries branch from the brachial artery at the elbow level. The radial artery continues down the forearm in line with the radius while the ulnar artery descends parallel to the ulna. Both arteries are located in the volar compartment of the forearm. When the radial and ulnar arteries reach the wrist, each divide into superficial and deep branches to form the superficial and deep palmar arterial arches. The ulnar artery pulse can be felt just radial to the volar surface of the pisiform while the radial artery is palpable radial to the flexor carpi radialis tendon at the wrist (Fig. 8-2).

Immediately distal to the pisiform, the ulnar artery divides within Guyon canal into superficial and deep branches. The superficial branch is larger and contributes to most of the superficial arterial arch. The smaller deep branch of the ulnar artery makes up the nondominant portion of the deep arterial arch. Just proximal to the pisiform, the ulnar artery gives off volar and dorsal branches that unite with similar branches from the radial artery to form the circumferential dorsal and palmar carpal arterial network that supplies the carpal bones. Perforating branches from the deep arch pass between the ring and the middle finger metacarpal bases to unite with the dorsal carpal arterial arch. Distal to this, the dorsal carpal arch sends dorsal metacarpal arteries that are located in the dorsal subaponeurotic space. These terminate in the dorsal digital arteries that end at the PIP joint level.

At the radial styloid, the radial artery divides into superficial and deep branches. The superficial branch continues either over or through the thenar eminence into the palm to complete the superficial palmar arch in most patients. Occasionally, the superficial arch is incomplete if the superficial branches of the radial and the

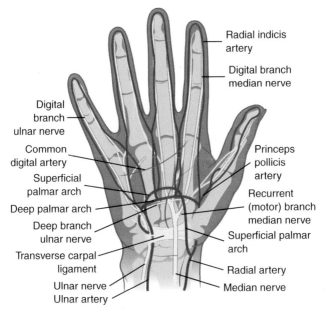

FIGURE 8-1 Arterial system of the hand.

ulnar arteries do not unite with one another. The deep branch of the radial artery is larger and dominates the deep arterial arch. It can be felt occasionally in the anatomical snuffbox where it passes underneath the tendons of the first and third dorsal compartments, which make up the boundaries of the anatomical snuffbox. The deep branch of the radial artery then passes between the two heads of the first dorsal interosseous muscle to reach the palm where it joins with the smaller deep branch of the ulnar artery to form the deep palmar arterial arch.

A line drawn across the ulnar border of the radially abducted thumb across the palm approximates the location of the superficial arterial arch. The deep arch is about 1 cm proximal and deep to the superficial arch. The superficial arch arterial diameter is larger and gives the predominant blood supply to the digits. However, if the superficial arch is damaged, the digits may still survive because of the collateral blood flow through the deep arch.

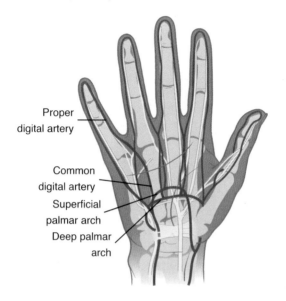

Proper digital artery

Common digital artery

Superficial palmar arch

Deep palmar arch

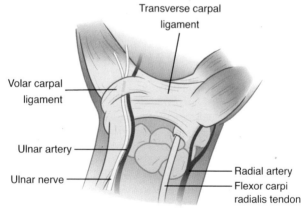

Transverse carpal ligament

Volar carpal ligament

Ulnar artery

Ulnar nerve

Radial artery

Flexor carpi radialis tendon

FIGURE 8-2 Radial and ulnar arteries at the wrist.

The superficial palmar arch branches into common digital vessels along the second, third, and fourth intermetacarpal areas termed common digital arteries. These arteries are located within the second, third, and fourth web space canals. The radial side of the index finger and the ulnar side of the small finger typically have their own individual branches which come off either the deep or superficial arch, respectively. Proximal to the web spaces, the common digital arteries then bifurcate into proper digital arteries to each of the neighboring sides of the digits. In the palm, these arteries are just deep to the palmar fascial complex but are superficial to the branches of the median and ulnar nerves. At the level where the common digital arteries bifurcate, the nerves become superficial (anterior) to the arteries. This relationship, nerve superficial to the artery, persists into the fingers. The palmar metacarpal arteries, which are branches of the deep arterial arch, unite with the common digital arteries, which are branches of the superficial arch just prior to the bifurcation of the common digital arteries into proper digital arteries. Each digit has two digital arteries, radial and ulnar, which are accompanied by a digital nerve superficial to it. Just proximal to the level of the PIP joint, the digital artery sends a dorsal branch to the dorsum of the finger to further supply the skin in this area. At the level of the DIP joint, the digital artery then divides into its three terminal branches which supply the tissue of the pulp and the nail bed. There are dorsal branches from the digital artery which supply the dorsal skin at the level of the DIP joint.

Similar to the arterial supply of the hand, there is a superficial and deep set of veins. The superficial veins are large and located in the dorsal subcutaneous space of the hand over the dorsal aponeurosis, which incorporates the extensor tendons. Fewer palmar veins that belong to the superficial venous system are also encountered and begin in the digits. Veins of the superficial system from both dorsal and palmar areas join the cephalic and basilic veins in the wrist area, which continue in the forearm. Deep venous drainage is coupled with the arterial system as small veins typically run contiguous with the arteries called venae comitantes.

The superficial venous system is the more dominant (Fig. 8-3) as it is larger than the deep system. The superficial veins are found in the loose areolar subcutaneous space primarily in the dorsum of the hand and digits. Gravity can be used to demonstrate the dorsal

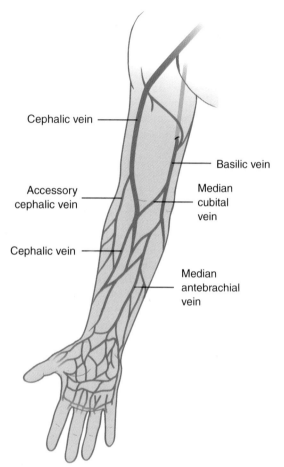

FIGURE 8-3 Upper extremity superficial venous system.

veins in the hand which become prominent when the hand is held by the side. The superficial venous system of the hand continues as the cephalic and basilic veins on the radial and ulnar borders of the wrist and forearm, respectively. Often, there is a third large vein on the central volar aspect of the wrist, the median antebrachial vein,

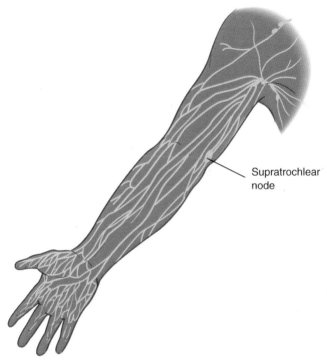

Supratrochlear
node

FIGURE 8-4 Upper extremity superficial lymphatic system.

which receives inflow from the smaller superficial palmar veins. The superficial and deep veins anastomose with each other by variable numbers of communicating or perforating veins at the palm and wrist.

The deep venous system of the hand has clinical relevance, especially in planning free flaps or tissue transfers for reconstructive hand surgery. The radial and ulnar arteries at the wrist are accompanied by venae comitantes, which are typically small paired veins contiguous with each artery. These companion veins are essential for facilitating venous outflow of surgically transferred soft tissue based on radial and ulnar arteries.

The lymphatic vessels accompany the veins in the hand and wrist. This is easy to understand when the same mesenchymal tissue is the basis for both veins and lymphatic vessels. There is both a superficial and deep set of lymphatic vessels which correspond to the superficial and deep venous systems. While some of the lymphatic drainage from the fingers will proceed toward the palm, most of the lymphatic drainage proceeds to the dorsal aspect of the hand. The lymphatics from the thenar and hypothenar areas of the hand tend to flow into the loose areolar tissue of the dorsal subcutaneous space. The dorsal hand swelling encountered with infections of the palmar aspect of the hand can be attributed to lymphedema. Once it reaches the wrist level, lymphatic fluid continues to drain in lymph vessels accompanying cephalic and basilic veins. It is through this lymphatic drainage that bacteria or tumor cells from the index finger or thumb have an easier access to the thoracic duct since the cephalic vein drains into this area. The lymphatic fluid from the hand drains to epitrochlear, axillary, and deltopectoral lymph nodes (Fig. 8-4). There are relatively few lymph nodes around the path of the basilic vein.

Peripheral Nervous System

Understanding the peripheral nervous system of the hand and upper extremity is critical to accurately diagnose and treat the various pathologies that are encountered in the upper limb. Knowing the anatomy is paramount to gaining that understanding. Surgical approaches of the upper limb require thorough knowledge of course and relationship of the nerves and their surrounding structures.

BRACHIAL PLEXUS

The brachial plexus is formed by the merger of C5-T1 nerve roots. It gives rise to multiple branches that coalesce and split to form the peripheral nerves of the upper extremity. The plexus is composed of five roots, three trunks, six divisions, three cords, and multiple branches (Fig. 9-1). The C5-T1 roots are formed by the dorsal and ventral rootlets as they exit the cervical spine. The dorsal root ganglion contains the cell bodies for the sensory nerves. Injuries to the brachial plexus are divided into preganglionic (spinal cord avulsions) and post-ganglionic (more peripheral injuries). Differentiating between these two categories is important and has treatment implications (Fig. 9-1).

ULNAR NERVE

The ulnar nerve arises from the medial cord of the brachial plexus with contributions from C8 and T1. It runs anterior to the triceps muscle in the upper arm and medial to the brachial artery. Approximately halfway down the arm it passes posteriorly and pierces the medial intermuscular septum to enter the posterior compartment of the arm. It then continues posterior to the medial epicondyle within the fibro-osseous compartment of the cubital

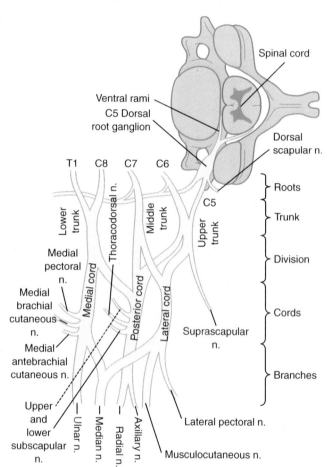

FIGURE 9-1 Anatomy of the brachial plexus.

tunnel to enter the forearm. The ulnar nerve has no branches in the arm.

At the elbow, the ulnar nerve passes between the two heads of the flexor carpi ulnaris (FCU) and accesses the forearm to run along the ulnar surface of the flexor digitorum profundus (FDP). It innervates

Ulnar nerve

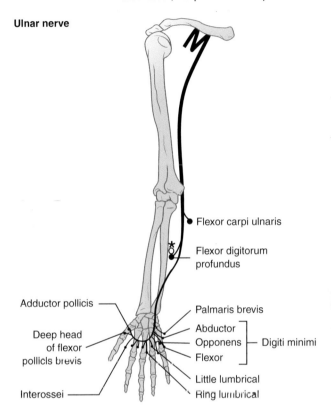

Flexor carpi ulnaris

Flexor digitorum profundus

Adductor pollicis

Deep head of flexor pollicis brevis

Interossei

Palmaris brevis

Abductor ⎤
Opponens ⎬ Digiti minimi
Flexor ⎦

Little lumbrical

Ring lumbrical

* Profundus muscle is also supplied by median nerve (see text)

FIGURE 9-2 The motor innervation of the ulnar nerve.

the FCU and FDP of the ring and small fingers. The motor innervation of the ulnar nerve is shown in Figure 9-2. At the mid-forearm, the ulnar artery runs with the nerve on its radial (lateral) side. Just proximal to the wrist, the ulnar nerve gives off the dorsal sensory branch of the ulnar nerve. This branch supplies sensation to the ulnar side of the palm, the ulnar side of the dorsal hand and the dorsal small finger, and the dorsal, ulnar half of the ring finger (Fig. 9-3).

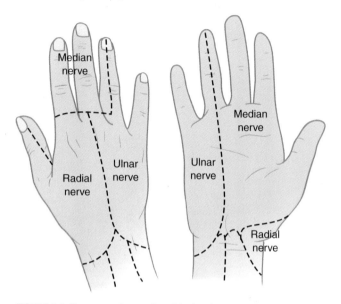

FIGURE 9-3 The sensory innervation of the hand.

At the wrist, the nerve runs within and deep to the FCU tendon, with the tendon most medial, the ulnar artery most lateral, and the nerve in between. It continues along the radial side of the pisiform into Guyon's canal. The borders of Guyon's canal are the pisiform (ulnar border), hamate (radial border), the transverse carpal ligament (floor), and volar carpal ligament (roof) (Fig. 9-4).

There are three zones through which the ulnar nerve passes at the wrist. In zone 1, the nerve consists of motor and sensory fibers that run together and is located ulnar to the ulnar artery. At the end of zone 1, the nerve bifurcates into the superficial sensory and deep motor branches. Zone II contains the deep motor branch of the ulnar nerve which supplies the following muscles: adductor pollicis, the third and fourth lumbricals, all seven interosseoi, the deep head of the flexor pollicis brevis, and the muscles of the hypothenar group—the palmaris brevis, the abductor digiti minimi, the flexor digiti minimi brevis, and the opponens digiti minimi. Zone 3 contains the sensory branch which gives rise to the digital nerves

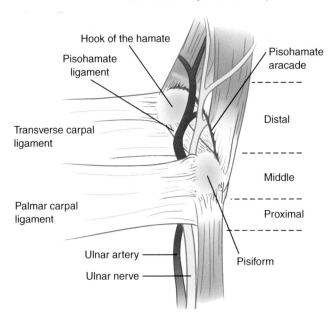

FIGURE 9-4 The anatomy of Guyon canal.

that supply the skin to the small finger and the ulnar digital nerve to the ring finger.

MEDIAN NERVE

The median nerve arises from the medial and lateral cords of the brachial plexus and has contributions from C5, C6, C7, C8, and T1. It runs along the radial side of the brachial artery in the arm until the mid-arm where it crosses the artery and runs along its ulnar side. It remains in the anterior compartment of the arm and distally it courses along the brachialis muscle. The median nerve has no branches in the arm.

At the elbow, the median nerve passes deep to the biceps aponeurosis and between the two heads of the pronator teres. Here the nerve innervates the pronator teres, the flexor carpi radialis, the palmaris longus, and the flexor digitorum superficialis. It gives off a

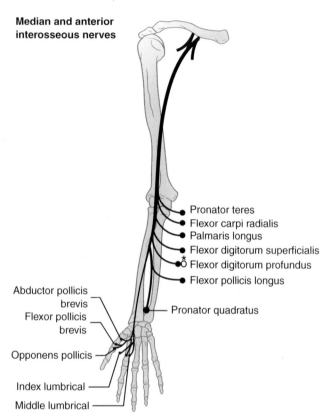

**Median and anterior
interosseous nerves**

Pronator teres
Flexor carpi radialis
Palmaris longus
Flexor digitorum superficialis
* Flexor digitorum profundus
Flexor pollicis longus

Abductor pollicis
brevis

Flexor pollicis
brevis

Pronator quadratus

Opponens pollicis

Index lumbrical

Middle lumbrical

* Profundus muscle is also supplied by
  ulnar nerve (see text)

FIGURE 9-5 The motor innervation of the median nerve.

branch, the anterior interosseus nerve (AIN). The AIN supplies the
radial half of the FDP, the flexor pollicis longus, and the pronator
quadrates. The AIN terminates in articular branches to the wrist
joint. The median nerve proper in the forearm is located between the
flexor digitorum superficialis and FDP muscle bellies. The motor
innervation of the median nerve is shown in Figure 9-5.

Approximately 5–7 centimeters proximal to the wrist, the palmar cutaneous branch of the median nerve arises from the radial side of the nerve. It courses superficial between the tendons of the flexor carpi radialis and palmaris longus muscles and supplies the skin of the radial palm and thenar eminence. The median nerve continues through the carpal tunnel with nine flexor tendons. The borders of the carpal tunnel are the carpometacarpal joints and carpal bones (floor and sides) and the transverse carpal ligament and its proximal extension, the flexor retinaculum (roof). At the distal edge of the carpal tunnel, the nerve divides into six branches: the common digital nerve to the third web space, the common digital nerve to the second web space, the radial digital nerve to the index finger, the ulnar digital nerve to the thumb, the radial digital nerve to the thumb, and the recurrent motor branch. The sensory innervations of the median nerve are to the volar thumb, and the dorsal and volar index finger, middle finger, and radial half of the ring finger (Fig. 9-3). The recurrent motor branch comes off the radial side of the median nerve and loops back proximally over the transverse carpal ligament to innervate the thenar musculature including the abductor pollicis brevis, the opponens pollicis, and a portion of the flexor pollicis brevis (with the ulnar nerve). There are also two small branches of the recurrent motor branch to the first and second lumbrical muscles.

RADIAL NERVE

The radial nerve is the largest terminal branch of the posterior cord and largest terminal nerve of the brachial plexus. It arises from the C5, C6, C7, C8, and T1 roots. The radial nerve exits the axilla through a triangular space between the long and medial heads of the triceps muscle and continues from medial to lateral along the posterior arm in the radial groove of the humerus. When it reaches the lateral humerus in passes anteriorly through the lateral intermuscular septum and travels between the brachialis and the brachioradialis muscles to the level of the lateral epicondyle. It gives branches to the triceps, anconeus, brachioradialis, and one half of the brachialis muscles in the arm. It often supplies the extensor carpi radialis longus.

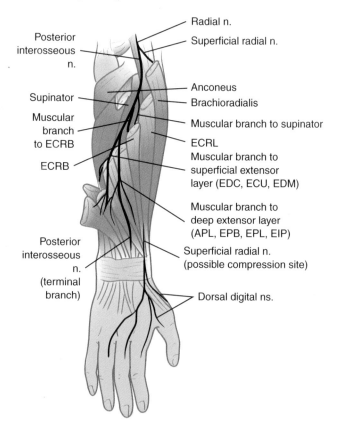

FIGURE 9-6 Anatomy of the posterior interosseous nerve. ECRL, extensor carpi radialis longus; ECRB, extensor carpi radialis brevis; EDC, extensor digitorum communis; ECU, extensor carpi ulnaris; APL, abductor pollicis longus; EPB, extensor pollicis brevis; EPL, extensor pollicis longus; EIP, extensor indicis proprius; EDM, extensor digiti minimi.

At the level of the radiocapitellar joint of the elbow, the nerve splits into the superficial radial nerve (which is purely sensory) and the posterior interosseous nerve (PIN), which is purely motor. The superficial radial nerve travels underneath the brachioradialis until it exits dorsally and becomes superficial in the

Radial and posterior interosseous nerves

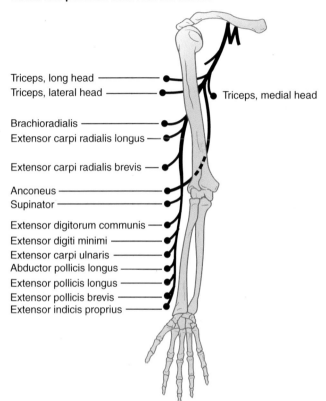

Triceps, long head
Triceps, lateral head
Triceps, medial head

Brachioradialis
Extensor carpi radialis longus

Extensor carpi radialis brevis

Anconeus
Supinator

Extensor digitorum communis
Extensor digiti minimi
Extensor carpi ulnaris
Abductor pollicis longus
Extensor pollicis longus
Extensor pollicis brevis
Extensor indicis proprius

FIGURE 9-7 The motor innervation of the radial nerve.

distal third of the forearm to supply the skin of the dorsal hand and thumb (Fig. 9-3).

The PIN (Fig. 9-6) can give a branch to the extensor carpi radialis longus or it can arise directly from the radial nerve. The PIN then passes between the superficial and deep heads of the supinator muscle (which it innervates). As it passes through the forearm, the PIN innervates the extensor carpi radialis brevis, extensor digitorum communis, extensor digiti minimi, extensor carpi ulnaris, abductor pollicis longus, extensor pollicis longus and brevis, and extensor indicis proprius. The motor innervation of the radial nerve is shown in Figure 9-7. It terminates by giving sensory branches to the dorsal wrist capsule.

Musculotendinous System

FLEXOR TENDONS

The three wrist flexor tendons pass anteriorly and outside of the carpal tunnel: the palmaris longus (PL), flexor carpi radialis, and flexor carpi ulnaris (FCU). The flexor carpi radialis attaches onto the base of the second metacarpal, the FCU attaches onto the pisiform and base of the fifth metacarpal, and the PL (the weakest of the three) distally becomes the palmar fascia. Approximately 20% of the population does not have a PL tendon. The FCU is the most powerful wrist flexor and provides the ulnar deviation force that is important in power gripping, as when using tools and hammering.

At the level of the wrist, the nine extrinsic (originating in the forearm) digital flexor tendons pass through the carpal tunnel. The four tendons of the flexor digitorum superficialis (FDS) are the most superficial. Each tendon of the FDS comes from a separate muscle belly, allowing independent digital proximal interphalangeal (PIP) joint flexion. The exception sometimes is the small finger, whose FDS tendon may have a cross-connection to the FDS of the ring finger. At the level of the forearm and wrist, the FDS tendons to the middle and ring fingers are superficial to those of the index and small fingers. One common way to remember this is that "34" is greater than "25." Each of the four FDS tendons inserts onto the volar surface of a finger's middle phalanx to produce PIP joint flexion. Each finger, except possibly the small, can be independently controlled by its FDS tendon. The four tendons of the flexor digitorum profundus (FDP) run deep to those of the FDS. Each FDP tendon inserts onto the volar surface of a finger's distal phalanx to produce distal interphalangeal (DIP) joint flexion. The FDP tendons to the middle, ring, and small digit all come from a single muscle belly, which prevents it from contributing to independent finger flexion, except for the index finger, which has an independent FDP muscle. The flexor pollicis longus tendon is the most radial structure in the carpal tunnel and attaches onto the base of the distal phalanx of the thumb to flex the interphalangeal (IP) joint.

Proximal to the metacarpophalangeal joints (MPJs), the extrinsic digital flexors enter a flexor sheath within a fibro-osseous tunnel. The purpose of this tunnel is to position the flexor tendons close to the bones in the finger to prevent them from "bowstringing" and to maximize the efficiency of the tendons in creating joint motion. The fibroserous sheath has a series of thickenings in it known as pulleys. The most important of these are the A2 pulley, which is over the proximal phalanx, and the A4 pulley, which is over the middle phalanx. The odd numbered pulleys (A1, A3, and A5) are located over joints (the MP, PIP, and DIP joints, respectively) (Fig. 10-1). Each tendon has two vincula, vincula brevis and longus, that contain vascular supply to the tendons (Fig. 10-2). At the level of the proximal phalanx the FDS divides into two slips, which pass on either side of the FDP tendon to form "Camper's chiasm." The hand is described to have five zones based on the anatomy of the flexor tendons. Zone

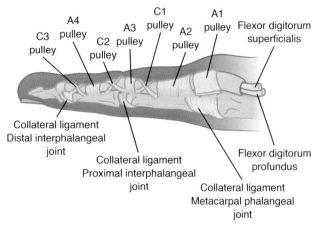

FIGURE 10-1 The flexor tendons with annular **(A)** and cruciate **(C)** pulleys. The cruciate pulleys are thinner areas between the annular pulleys that fold up with digital flexion A, annular; C, cruciate; VLS, vincula longus superficialis; B, brevis; P, profondus.

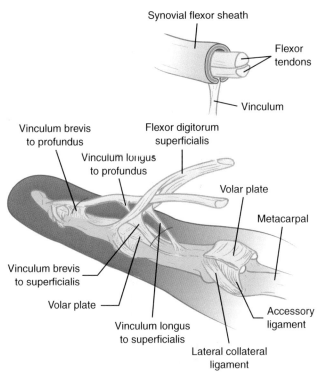

FIGURE 10-2 The vincula brevis and longus and the flexor digitorum profundus tendon passes through Camper chiasm in the flexor digitorum superficialis tendon at the level of the proximal phalanx.

II is the most distinguished as it contains both FDS and FDP tendons within the tendon sheath (Fig. 10-3).

EXTENSOR TENDONS

The digital extensor tendons in the wrist pass under the extensor retinaculum in six separate dorsal compartments (Fig. 10-4). Similar to the digital fibro-osseous tunnel, the extensor retinaculum holds the extensor tendons close to the bones to prevent "bowstringing" during combined hand and wrist extension, which would decrease

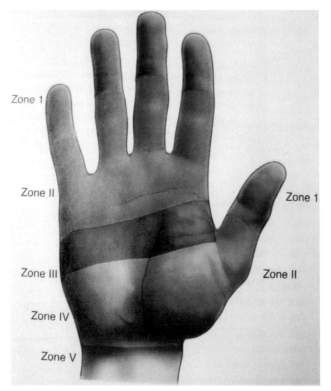

FIGURE 10-3 The five zones of the hand based on flexor tendon anatomy. Zone I contains flexor digitorum profundus tendon; zone II is the tendon sheath containing flexor digitorum superficialis and flexor digitorum profundus tendons; zone III is the lumbrical muscle zone, zone IV is the carpal tunnel region; and zone V is the forearm area. (From Wiesel, *Operative Techn Orth Surg.*, p. 2570).

the amount of joint motion that a given tendon excursion would produce.

The first dorsal compartment contains the tendons of the abductor pollicis longus (APL) and extensor pollicis brevis (EPB). The APL inserts on the base of the first metacarpal. Its role to abduct the thumb and aids in radially deviating the wrist. In 60% of

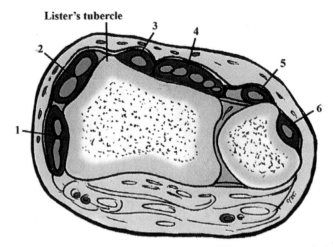

FIGURE 10-4 The six dorsal compartments of the extensor tendons. The abductor pollicis longus and extensor pollicis brevis pass through the first compartment. The extensor carpi radialis longus and extensor carpi radialis brevis pass through the second compartment. The extensor pollicis longus passes through the third compartment. The extensor digitorum communis and extensor indicis pass through the fourth compartment. The extensor digiti minimi pass through the fifth compartment. The extensor carpi ulnaris passes through the sixth compartment. (From HSU IV ASSH publication).

the population, there is a separate subcompartment for the EPB, which predisposes the EPB to entrapment, as in DeQuervain syndrome. The EPB inserts onto the base of the thumb's proximal phalanx its main role is to extend the MP joint of the thumb.

The second dorsal compartment contains the tendons of the extensor carpi radialis longus and the extensor carpi radialis brevis, both of which are powerful wrist extensors that insert onto the bases of the index and middle finger metacarpals, respectively.

The third dorsal compartment contains the extensor pollicis longus (EPL) tendon, which inserts onto the base of the thumb's distal phalanx and extends the IP joint. In addition, the EPL is the only tendon that allows for IP joint hyperextension and retropulsion of the thumb (bringing the thumb dorsal to the plane of the palm).

Together, the first and third compartment tendons form the boundaries of the anatomic "snuff box."

The fourth dorsal compartment contains the tendons of the extensor digitorum communis (EDC) and extensor indicis proprius (EIP). The EDC tendons insert into the extensor hood of all four fingers. The EIP attaches to the extensor hood of the index finger ulnar to the EDC of the index finger. At the level of the metacarpals, the EDC tendons [but not the EIP or extensor digiti minimi (EDM) tendons] are attached by junctura tendinae In the event of laceration of one EDC tendon, the junctura tendinae allow for weak digital extension of that digit. The junctura tendinae are more substantial and stronger on the ulnar side of the hand; for the majority of the population, the EDC contribution to the small finger consists of only a juncturae tendinae from the ringer finger, without a separate EDC tendon.

The fifth dorsal compartment contains the EDM tendon, which inserts into the small finger's dorsal hood on its ulnar side and blends with the EDC tendon of that finger. This tendon is often bifid (i.e., is made up of two separate smaller tendons).

The sixth dorsal compartment contains the tendon of the extensor carpi ulnaris, which is a powerful wrist extensor and ulnar deviator that attaches onto the base of the fifth metacarpal.

It is important to note that the extrinsic tendons' main function is to extend the MPJ, as the intrinsic muscles flex this joint. Counter-intuitively there is no actual anatomic insertion of the extrinsic tendons (or the flexor tendons) onto the proximal phalanx. The extrinsic tendon extends the MPJ through the sagittal bands on either side, which wrap around the base of the proximal phalanx and attach in a soft tissue confluence near the palmar plate aiding in this joint extension. The sagittal bands stabilize the extrinsic tendons from either side and prevent their lateral subluxation, which would compromise their ability to extend this joint. The hand is described to have seven zones based on the anatomy of the extensor tendons (Fig. 10-5).

INTRINSIC MUSCLES

The term intrinsic implies that the muscles both originate and insert within the hand. The intrinsic muscles of the hand include

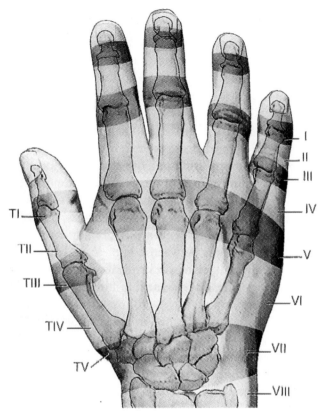

FIGURE 10-5 The seven zones of the hand based on extensor tendon anatomy. The odd zones I, III, V, and VII belong to distal interphalangeal, proximal interphalangeal, metacarpophalangeal, and wrist joints, respectively. The even zones II, IV, and VI belong to P2, P1, and metacarpal. (From Wiesel, *Operative Techn Orth Surg*, p. 2577).

the interosseous muscles (both volar and dorsal), the lumbricals, and the muscles of the thenar and hypothenar eminences.

Interosseous Muscles

The four dorsal interossei origin called Interosseous Muscles originate from the metacarpals and insert via two tendons: one

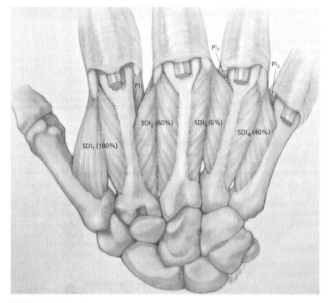

FIGURE 10-6 The four dorsal interossei provide finger abduction. The numbers indicate the percentages of tendon insertion in the proximal phalanx as oppose to extensor hood mechanism. (Adapted from Doyle and Botte, *Surgical Anatomy*, Fig 10.38, p. 584).

into the proximal phalanx, where they provide abduction of the fingers, and one into the extensor mechanism (Fig. 10-6). The three volar interossei originate from the metacarpals and insert into the lateral bands of the extensor hood to provide adduction of the fingers (Fig. 10-7). It is easy to remember which interossei abduct and adduct the fingers by simply observing that fingers extend (move dorsally) slightly with abduction and flex (move volarly) slightly with adduction. The small finger does not have a dorsal interosseous muscle. This finger abduction is provided by the abductor digiti quinti (ADQ), one of the hypothenar muscles. The small finger is adducted by the third volar interosseous and, unlike the thumb, does not have a separate adductor muscle.

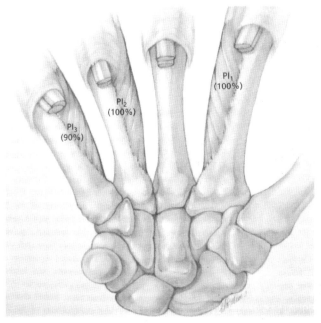

FIGURE 10-7 The three volar interossei provide finger adduction. The percentages indicate that the tendons almost always insert in the extensor hood mechanism. (Adapted from Doyle and Botte, *Surgical Anatomy*, Fig 10.40, p. 586).

Lumbrical Muscles

The lumbricals are the only muscles in the body to both originate from and insert onto a tendon. They originate from the FDP tendon and insert onto the radial lateral bands of the extensor hoods. The lumbrical muscles of the index and middle fingers originate from their respective FDP tendons and course radially through the "lumbrical canal," volar to the axis of the MPJ. The lumbrical muscles of the ring and small fingers originate from two adjacent FDP tendons (the third and fourth, and the fourth and fifth, respectively) before passing through their lumbrical canals.

The extensor hood or mechanism of each finger spans the MP and DIP joints. It is a blending of the extrinsic extensor tendons (the EDC, EIP, and EDM) and the intrinsic tendons (the interossei

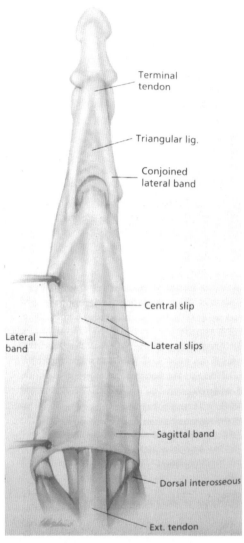

FIGURE 10-8 Dorsal view of the extensor hood and the intrinsic muscles. (Adapted from Doyle and Botte, *Surgical Anatomy*, Fig 10.43, p. 590).

and lumbricals) (Fig. 10-8). The mid-point of the extensor mechanism is a tendinous extension that attaches onto the base of the middle phalanx (called the central tendon or slip) and produces extension of the PIP joint. At the level of the proximal phalanx, the extensor tendons also give off the lateral bands on either side that merge with the intrinsic tendons over the middle phalanx to form the terminal tendon, which inserts onto the base of the distal phalanx to produce extension of the DIP joint.

By joining the extrinsic extensor system on both sides of the digit, the intrinsic tendons therefore aid in PIP joint extension through the central tendon and DIP joint extension through the terminal tendon.

The tendons of the intrinsic muscles pass volar to the axis of MPJ rotation and dorsal to the axis of the PIP and DIP joints' centers of rotation. Therefore, the intrinsic muscles flex the MPJs and extend both the PIP and the DIP joints. Despite the fact that the extrinsic tendon system contributes to both the central slip and the terminal tendon, PIP and DIP joint extension is primarily a function of the intrinsic system.

The lateral bands have restraining ligaments that provide them sagittal (volar–dorsal) stability, similar to how the sagittal bands maintain the extrinsic extensor tendons centered over the MPJ. The triangular ligament joins the two lateral bands together dorsally over the middle phalanx and prevents their volar subluxation. The transverse retinacular ligament originates from the flexor sheaths and attaches to the lateral bands volarly at the level of the PIP joint and prevents their dorsal subluxation.

Thenar Muscles

The thenar muscles are a group of three muscles at the base of the thumb: the abductor pollicis brevis (APB), opponens pollicis, and flexor pollicis brevis (FPB). All three muscles take origin from the transverse carpal ligament and the trapezium. The APB is superficial and radial; it abducts the thumb out of the palm (i.e., palmar abduction), which is a key component of thumb opposition. It inserts onto the radial side of the proximal phalanx and MPJ. The FPB is located volar and ulnar, allowing it to flex the thumb MPJ. The FPB has two heads that are split by the flexor pollicis longus; the superficial head inserts onto the radial side of the proximal phalanx. The deep head originates from the thumb metacarpal (a partial exception to the aforementioned origins) and inserts into the ulnar side of the proximal phalanx; each tendinous insertion is associated with a sesamoid bone. The opponens pollicis is deep to both the APB and the FPB muscles. It is the only thenar muscle that attaches onto the thumb metacarpal to aid its flexion at the TM joint.

The adductor pollicis is not considered one of the thenar muscles. Its transverse head arises from the middle finger metacarpal and its oblique head arises from the bases of the index and middle metacarpals. Both heads insert onto the base of the thumb's proximal phalanx and its ulnar sesamoid. The adductor pollicis provides power for key pinch as when turning a key or peeling open a packet.

Hypothenar Muscles

The hypothenar muscles mirror those of the thenar mass, consisting of three muscles at the base of the small finger. They include the ADQ, flexor digit quinti, and opponens digiti quinti. The superficial ADQ abducts the small finger. It takes origin from the pisiform and inserts into the proximal phalanx of the small finger. The flexor digit quinti is more central (radial) than the ADQ, similar to the way that the FDB is more central than the APB of the thumb. It flexes the small finger's MPJ. It takes origin from the hook of the hamate and inserts onto the proximal phalanx. Similar to the thumb, the opponens muscle is deepest and flexes the fifth metacarpal at its CMC joint during gripping. It originates from the body of the hamate and inserts onto the fifth metacarpal.

11

Retinacular System

The term retinaculum is derived from the Latin verb "retinere." By definition, a retinacular structure is a fibrous band that either stabilizes or retains skin and especially tendons in place. Retinacula are critically important in the function of the hand and wrist. Without their structural integrity normal tendon motion would be disturbed and joint and finger motion would be compromised.

Retinacular structures can be grouped into

- flexor retinacular complex of the wrist
- extensor retinaculum of the wrist
- digital flexor pulley system
- retinacular assembly of the extensor mechanism
- deep retinacular structures of the hand
- retaining ligaments of the skin.

FLEXOR RETINACULAR COMPLEX OF THE WRIST

The flexor and extensor retinacula are not continuous with each other. The flexor retinacular complex is a composite structure that consists of the flexor retinaculum, which is located in the distal forearm and continues with the antebrachial fascia, transverse carpal ligament (TCL), and the interthecal fascia between thenar and hypothenar areas.

The TCL (Fig. 11-1) originates from the carpal bones and forms the roof of the carpal canal. On the radial side, the retinaculum is attached to the scaphoid tubercle and the volar ridge of the trapezium. On the ulnar side, it blends into the pisotriquetral articulation proximally and firmly attaches to the hook of the hamate distally. These firm attachments contribute to the arcade

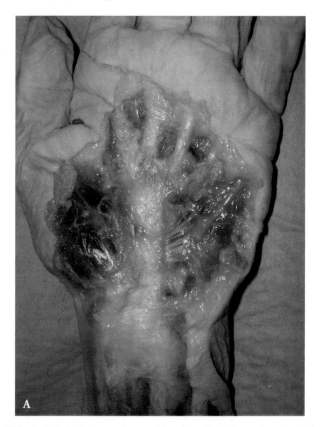

FIGURE 11-1 Cadaver specimen with palmar fascial complex removed, showing the three components of the flexor retinacular complex with the transverse carpal ligament as a narrow band in the middle giving origin to thenar and hypothenar muscles (**A**) and an illustration of the same area (Picture is courtesy of Ghazi Rayan MD) (*continued*)

configuration of the carpus in a manner similar to the string of a bow. The superficial surface of the TCL provides thenar muscle attachments radially, a passageway for the palmaris longus (PL) tendon centrally, and the floor for Guyon's canal ulnarly. The deep surface of the TCL allows the flexor tendons and median nerve to

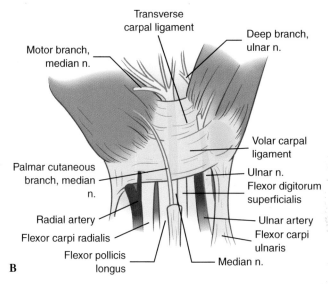

FIGURE 11-1 (*Continued*) (**B**) (Adaptation from HSU 3, p. 300, Fig. 1).

slide freely against its smooth surface. Proximally, the TCL blends with the flexor retinaculum of the forearm and distally, it blends into the fascia connecting the thenar and hypothenar fascia.

EXTENSOR RETINACULUM OF THE WRIST

The extensor retinaculum is directly attached to medial aspect of the ulna and lateral border of the radius (Fig. 11-2). It differs from the flexor retinaculum in that it has multiple fascial extensions from its deep surface that attach to bone and forms six compartments that hold the extensor tendons. The extensor retinaculum has six compartments. Occasionally the first dorsal compartment has a septum that separates the extensor pollicis brevis from the abductor pollicis longus; hence theoretically these patients have seven compartments. The extensor retinaculum distal margin attaches to the radio-carpal joint, and its deep surface is smooth to allow tendon gliding.

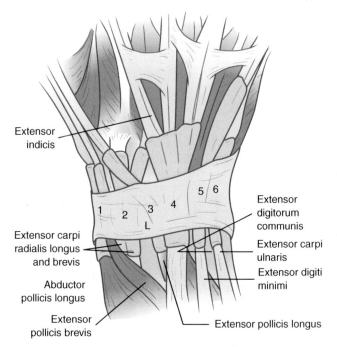

FIGURE 11-2 The wrist extensor retinaculum with six compartments. (Adaptation from Doyle and Botte, p. 648, Fig. 10.89).

FLEXOR PULLEY SYSTEM

The flexor pulley system overlies the flexor tendons and extends from the metacarpal neck to the base of the distal phalanx. It consists of a series of annular and cruciate pulleys. This system maintains the flexor tendons in proximity to bone and near the joint center of rotation, thereby enabling the greatest arc of motion with the most efficient tendon excursion during muscle contraction. Loss of one pulley following injury is not critical so long as the adjacent pulleys are intact. Loss of multiple pulleys leads to bowstringing of the tendons, reduces tendon excursion, and decreases joint motion. The two most important pulleys are the A2 and A4 pulleys. These two pulleys arise from and directly reattach to bone in the mid-portion of P1 (A2) and P2 (A4). The A2 pulley constrains both the flexor digitorum profundus and flexor digitorum superficialis tendons. In contrast, the A4 pulley proximal margin is over the flexor digitorum superficialis insertion of the P2 and thus only the flexor digitorum profundus is constrained and guided by it.

RETINACULAR ASSEMBLY OF THE EXTENSOR MECHANISM

These are a group of fascial bands that retain and stabilize the extrinsic extensor tendon over the metacarpophalangeal (MP) and proximal interphalangeal (PIP) joints and hence maximize these joints' function. Because of their retaining function and relationship to the intrinsic system their integrity is important for preventing collapse deformities of these joints.

- Sagittal band: The extensor mechanism is constrained at the level of the MP joint by the fibers of the sagittal bands (Fig. 11-3). These are essential for maintaining the central location of the extensor mechanism. The sagittal band fibers also augment the function of the extensor digitorum communis tendon to extend the MP joint. These fibers run superficial to the intrinsic muscle-tendon tissues as they insert in the soft tissue confluence near the palmar aspect of the MP joint. This allows the sagittal band to maintain stability of the extensor digitorum communis over the MP joint and metacarpal head while allowing proximal and distal excursion of the tendon. Sagittal band independence from the dorsal MP joint capsule is important for unimpeded motion of that joint.

- Transverse retinacular ligament: It consists of a thin fibrous sheet originating from the flexor tendon sheath and the PIP joint capsule palmar and inserts on the lateral border of the lateral bands dorsally (Fig. 11-4). It prevents dorsal subluxation of the lateral band during PIP joint extension.

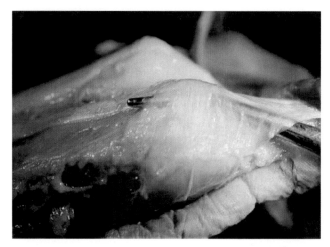

FIGURE 11-3 Anatomical specimen showing the sagittal band at the metacarpophalangeal joint level. (Picture is courtesy of Ghazi Rayan MD).

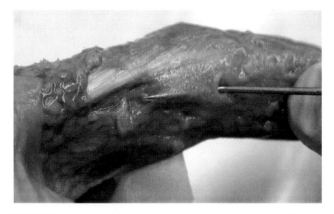

FIGURE 11-4 Anatomical specimen showing the transverse retinacular ligament at the proximal interphalangeal joint level. (Picture is courtesy of Ghazi Rayan MD).

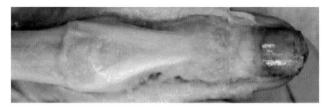

FIGURE 11-5 Anatomical specimen showing the central tendon at the proximal interphalangeal joint level and the terminal tendon at the distal interphalangeal joint level and triangular ligament between the lateral bands. (Picture is courtesy of Ghazi Rayan MD).

- Oblique retinacular ligament: This ligament is not easily identified and believed to be located deep to the transverse retinacular ligament and connect the fibrous sheath at the PIP joint level to the terminal tendon distal to the lateral band.
- Triangular ligament: This retinacular ligament is located between the radial and ulnar lateral bands (Fig. 11-5) immediately distal to the central tendon insertion in P2. It prevents palmar subluxation of the lateral bands during PIP joint flexion.

DEEP RETINACULAR STRUCTURES OF THE HAND

This consists of the three interpalmar plate ligaments, eight septa of Leugue and Juvara, and the soft tissue confluences located on each side of the MP joints (Chapter 6).

RETAINING LIGAMENTS OF THE SKIN

Skin stability during digital joint motion is important for hand function. Without fibrous tissue attachment between the digital skin and the underlying tissue, there would be minimal skin stability. Hand functions such as grabbing a knife or hammer would be difficult. Two fibrous tethers anchor the skin to deeper structures at the PIP and DIP joints, thereby stabilizing it on each side of the finger. Cleland ligament fibers course dorsal to the neurovascular bundle and Grayson ligament course volar to the

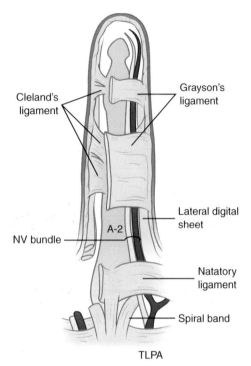

TLPA

FIGURE 11-6 An illustration of the Grayson ligament volar to the neurovascular bundle and Cleland ligament dorsal (reflected) to the neurovascular bundle. (Adaptation from Doyle and Botte, p. 620, Fig. 10.70).

same bundle (Fig. 11-6). The combined effect of these two ligaments provide stable positioning of the skin and neurovascular bundle during digital joint movement. The multiple small fibrous bands that are scattered in the volar aspect of the palm and digits also provide stability for the dermis during pinch and grasp (Chapter 6).

CHAPTER 12

Syndesmotic System

WRIST JOINT LIGAMENTS

The wrist is the most complicated joint in the human body. It contains 15 bones that contribute to its formation including 2 forearm bones, 8 carpal bones, and 5 metacarpal bones. Wrist joint articulations can be grouped into radiocarpal, midcarpal, interosseous, and distal radioulnar.

Multiple ligaments connect the bones of the radiocarpal joint. These ligaments are intracapsular (intra-articular) except for two outside the wrist capsule, the transverse carpal ligament, which forms the roof of the carpal tunnel and the pisohamate and piso-metacarpal ligaments. The intracapsular ligaments are difficult to distinguish when surgically approaching the joint. By contrast, when viewed from inside the joint with an arthroscope, the intra-capsular ligaments can be clearly identified.

INTRACAPSULAR LIGAMENTS

Intracapsular ligaments can be grouped into extrinsic and intrinsic ligaments. Extrinsic ligaments (Fig. 12-1 and 12-2) connect the distal radius and ulna to the carpal bones (carpus), whereas the intrinsic ligaments originate and insert within the carpus. Anatomic, histologic, and biochemical differences exist between these two groups. The extrinsic ligaments are stiffer but with lower yield strength than the intrinsic ligaments. The intrinsic ligaments have a relatively larger area of insertion into cartilage than into bone and contain less elastic fibers as compared with the extrinsic ligaments. They have different modes of failure under stress: The extrinsic ligaments tend to sustain mid-substance ruptures, whereas the intrinsic ligaments are more frequently avulsed than ruptured.

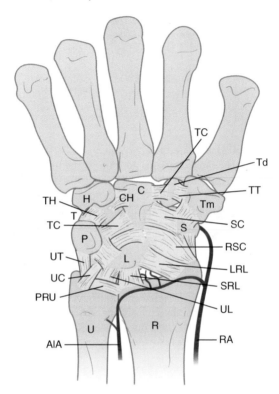

FIGURE 12-1 Palmar radiocarpal and ulnocarpal ligaments (From Hand Surgery Update #4, p. 272).

Extrinsic ligaments may be subdivided into three major groups: palmar radiocarpal, palmar ulnocarpal, and dorsal radiocarpal ligaments. There are no dorsal ligaments between the ulna and the carpus.

There are four volar ligaments that connect the radius to the carpus: the radioscaphoid, radioscaphoid-capitate, long radiolunate, and short radiolunate ligaments progressing from the radial styloid to the ulnar aspect of the distal radius. The first three ligaments originate from the radial third of the palmar margin of the distal radius and take an oblique course to insert into the

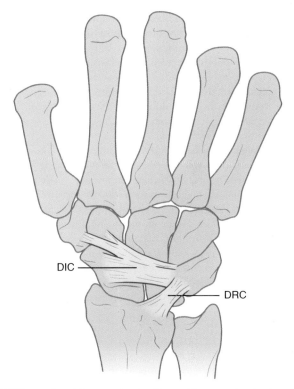

FIGURE 12-2 Dorsal intercarpal and radiocarpal ligaments forming lateral V with the apex at the triquetrum (From Hand Surgery Update #4, p. 272).

scaphoid tuberosity (radioscaphoid), the volar aspect of the capitate (radioscaphoid-capitate), and the lunate (long radiolunate). The short radiolunate ligament originates from the ulnar anterior rim of the radius and has a vertical direction inserting into the volar aspect of the lunate. The radioscaphoid-capitate ligament courses around the palmar concavity of the scaphoid, forming a hinge over which the scaphoid rotates. Between the two diverging radioscaphoid-capitate and long radiolunate ligaments, there is an area named the space of Poirier. This space represents a weak zone through which perilunate dislocations of the carpus frequently occur. In many instances, the long radiolunate ligament appears to be in continuity with the intrinsic lunate triquetrum interosseous ligament (LTIL) at its volar margin. The so-called radioscaphoid-lunate ligament, for a long time considered a deep intracapsular ligament, is not a true ligament but a collection of disorganized loose connective tissue-containing vessels supplying the scapholunate interosseous ligament (SLIL) and adjacent osseous structures.

From the base of the ulnar styloid, called the fovea, the ulnocapitate ligament attaches to the neck of the capitate. The distal insertions of the ulnocapitate and radioscaphoid-capitate ligaments form the arcuate ligament, which has an inverted V_ shape. Dorsal to the ulnocapitate ligament, arising from the dorsal rim of the triangular fibrocartilage complex, are the ulnotriquetral and ulnolunate ligaments, which insert distally on the anterior aspect of the lunate and triquetrum. These ligaments and the superficial ulnocapitate ligament form the ulnocarpal ligamentous complex. The ulnocarpal and radiolunate ligaments form the proximal V_ of the palmar ligamentous complex. Hence the palmar extrinsic ligaments can be thought of as opposing V_ shapes with the central area being the space of Poirier.

Dorsal Wrist Ligaments

There are two dorsal wrist ligaments: the dorsal radiocarpal and dorsal intercarpal ligaments. Both attach to the triquetrum and form a lateral V configuration. The dorsal radiocarpal ligament is also known as the dorsal radial triquetral ligament. It is a wide, fan-shaped ligament that connects the dorsal edge of the distal articular surface of the radius to the dorsal rim of the triquetrum, with some deep fibers inserting onto the lunate and rarely onto the scaphoid.

Intrinsic Carpal Ligaments

Intrinsic carpal ligaments also known as interosseous ligaments are collections of relatively short dorsal and palmar fibers that connect the bones of the same carpal row (palmar and dorsal interosseous ligaments) or link the two rows together radial and ulnar (Fig. 12-3).

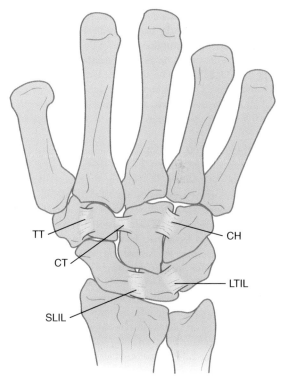

FIGURE 12-3 Interosseous ligaments (From Hand Surgery Update #4, p. 273).

The SLIL consists of three parts—the dorsal and volar scapholunate ligaments separated by a third, the fibrocartilaginous membrane. The dorsal scapholunate portion connects the dorsal-distal corners of the scaphoid and lunate bones. It is consists of thick fibers that play a key role in scapholunate stability. The palmar scapholunate portion allows more rotation and plays a lesser role in carpal stability. The membranous portion does not contribute to stability.

The LTIL has volar and dorsal components, and between the two there is a fibrocartilaginous membrane. In contrast to the SLIL, the volar lunate triquetral portion is thicker and stronger than the dorsal portion. Unless perforated by age or injury, this proximal membrane is a barrier between the radiocarpal and the midcarpal joint spaces. The fibers of the two portions of the LTIL are tighter through all ranges of motion than those of the SLIL, allowing little motion between the two bones. The most distal fibers of palmar and dorsal portions of LTIL are often connected to the distal fibers of the scapholunate joint. This may contribute to the stability of the luno-capitate joint by providing some enhancement to the depth of the midcarpal fossa but also provides stability to the scapholunate joint.

Midcarpal Ligaments

The dorsal intercarpal ligament arises from the dorsal ridge of the triquetrum, courses transversely along the distal edge of the lunate, and fans out to insert on the dorsal rim of the scaphoid, trapezium, and trapezoid bones. This structure may provide a stabilizing role to the lunocapitate joint. On the palmar side, the midcarpal joint is crossed by numerous ligaments. Ulnarly, a group of thick fibers connects the triquetrum to the hamate and capitate. This is known as the ulnar arm of the arcuate ligament. Laterally, the scaphoid tuberosity is linked to the distal row by two groups of fascicles: the anteromedial scaphoid capitate ligament and the dorsolateral Scapho-Trapezial-Trapezoid (STT) ligament. These ligaments are very important in the maintenance of the scaphoid normal alignment.

The existence of true radial and ulnar collateral ligaments of the wrist has been debated. The presence of very well-oriented collateral ligaments would constrain the wrist's extraordinary arc of motion.

Distal Carpal Row Interosseous Ligaments

The distal carpal row bones have numerous strong and taut transverse interosseous ligaments (dorsal, palmar, and deep intra-articular). They are particularly important in the protection of the carpal tunnel contents by maintaining the transverse carpal arch when compressive forces are applied.

Triangular Fibro Cartilage Complex

This complex has been described to have six components: dorsal and palmar radioulnar ligaments, articular disc, meniscus homologue, extensor carpi ulnaris subsheath, and ill-defined ulnar collateral ligament (Fig. 12-4).

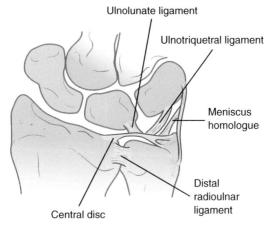

FIGURE 12-4 The components of the triangular fibrocartilage complex.

HAND LIGAMENTS

Carpometacarpal Joints

Dorsal and palmar intermetacarpal ligaments stabilize the inter-metacarpal joints. They consist of dorsal and palmar ligaments, which connect the base of each metacarpal to the corresponding surface of the distal carpal bone. Due to the strong nature of these ligaments, their injury is somewhat rare with the exception of the border digits—the thumb and small finger. These are the most mobile of the CMC joints with the thumb joint being the most mobile in the hand. The articular surfaces of the carpometacarpal joint of the thumb, which is termed trapeziometacarpal (TM) joint, resemble two reciprocally opposed saddles whose transverse axes are perpendicular. The TM joint has motion in three planes: flexion–extension, abduction–adduction, and pronation–supination (or opposition–retropulsion). There are four major ligaments: volar (anterior oblique), intermetacarpal, dorsal-radial, and dorsal oblique (posterior oblique). The volar oblique ligament, which connects the trapezium to the volar beak of the thumb metacarpal, is the primary restraint to dorsal subluxation force, which is inherent with pinch.

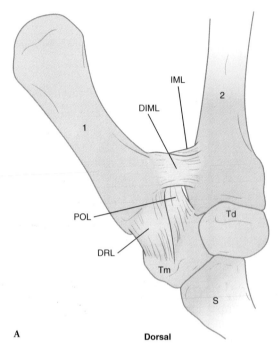

FIGURE   12-5 Dorsal   trapeziometacarpal   ligaments   (**A**)   and   palmar rapeziometacarpal ligaments (*continued*)

Metacarpophalangeal Joints

The metacarpal head is narrow dorsally and wider volarly giving progressively more contact with the base of the proximal phalanx with increasing flexion. The capsule of the metacarpophalangeal (MP) joint extends from the metacarpal neck to the base of the proximal phalanx and is reinforced with specialized structures on all sides. The capsule is composed of areolar tissue dorsally. On the volar side, the joint is supported by the palmar plate, which is continuous laterally with the interpalmar plate ligament. The palmar plate has a thick fibrocartilaginous distal portion and a thin membranous proximal portion. Lateral reinforcement for the palmar plate is afforded by the collateral and accessory collateral

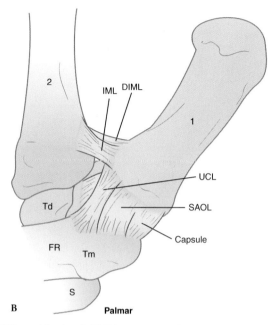

FIGURE 12-5 (*Continued*) (**B**) TM joint ligaments (From Doyle and Botte, p. 539.)

ligaments. The accessory collateral ligament inserts into the lateral margin of the palmar plate on both sides to produce a linked ligament-box support from one MP joint to another by the interpalmar plate ligament. The sagittal bands and the tendons of the intrinsic muscles provide additional secondary support.

The collateral ligaments have eccentric dorsal attachments to the metacarpal head. These ligaments are more taught in flexion than in extension because of the cam effect created by both the ligament attachment and shape of the metacarpal head which has a longer dorsal–volar axis (Fig. 12-6). There is broader and more stable articular contact between the metacarpal head and the base of the proximal phalanx beyond 70 degrees of flexion. The joint is stable laterally in full flexion but allows abduction and adduction in full extension.

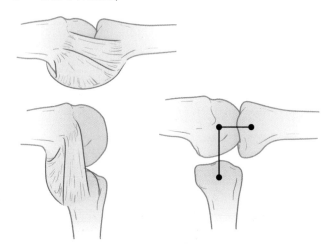

FIGURE 12-6 The collateral ligaments of the MP joint have eccentric dorsal attachments into the metacarpal head and are more taught in flexion than in extension. (From Rockwood and Green, p. 659, Fig. 11–53, 4th edition.)

Interphalangeal Joints

The ligamentous anatomy of the proximal interphalangeal (PIP) and distal interphalangeal joints is different, but their bony anatomy is similar. The IP joint is a hinge joint with stability from its bony articular contours, the collateral ligaments, and the palmar plate.

The PIP joint collateral ligaments arise from a concave fossa on the lateral aspect of each condyle and pass obliquely and volarly to their insertions. The collateral ligaments have proper and volar accessory collateral components. They are anatomically confluent but distinguished by their points of insertion. The proper collateral ligament inserts on the volar one-third base of the middle phalanx, whereas the accessory collateral ligament inserts on the palmar plate. The collateral ligaments are the primary restraints to radial and ulnar joint stress.

The palmar plate forms the floor of the joint and is suspended laterally by the collateral ligaments. The thick fibrocartilaginous distal portion inserts across the volar base of the middle phalanx. This insertion is only densely attached at its lateral margins, where it is confluent with the insertion of the collateral ligament. Centrally it blends with the volar periosteum of the middle phalanx. Laterally,

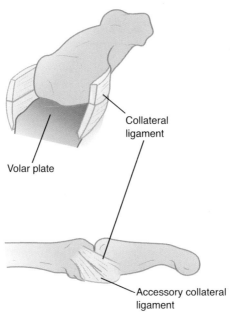

FIGURE 12-7 PIP joint has a boxlike complex that is secured laterally by the collateral ligaments and volarly by the palmar plate.

the palmar plate thickens to form a pair of proximal extensions called checkrein ligaments. The checkrein ligaments originate from the periosteum of the proximal phalanx, just inside the walls of the second annular (A2) pulley at its distal margin and are confluent with the proximal origins of the first cruciate (C1) pulley. These ligaments prevent hyperextension of the joint, while permitting full flexion. The palmar plate is a secondary stabilizer against lateral deviation when the collateral ligaments are incompetent or torn.

The key to PIP joint stability is the boxlike complex that is well secured laterally by the collateral ligaments and volarly by the palmar plate (Fig. 12-7). This configuration produces a three-dimensional structure that resists PIP joint displacement. For dislocation of the joint to occur, this ligament complex must be disrupted in at least two planes. Typically, collateral ligaments fail proximally, and the palmar plate avulses distally.

CHAPTER 13

Osseous Anatomy of the Hand and Wrist Biomechanics

THE HAND

The hand is compromised of five digits, four fingers, and a thumb. To facilitate communication between medical professionals the names of the fingers have been standardized as index, middle (long), ring, and small fingers.

The bones of each finger consist of (from proximal to distal) the following: the metacarpal, the proximal phalanx (P1), the middle phalanx (P2), and the distal phalanx (P3). The thumb has only two phalanges: the proximal (P1) and distal (P2) phalanges (Fig. 13-1). Each of these bones has ligamentous attachments and some provide muscle origins or tendinous insertions.

These bones contribute to the formation of the digital joints. Each finger has three joints: the metacarpophalangeal (MP) joint formed by the metacarpal and P1, the proximal interphalangeal (PIP) joint formed by P1 and P2, and the distal interphalangeal (DIP) joint formed by P2 and P3. The interphalangeal joints (i.e., the DIP and PIP joints) are hinge joints and allow only flexion and extension. They have thick collateral ligaments on either side that prevent side-to-side motion (i.e., radial or ulnar deviation). The collateral ligaments of the PIP and DIP joints are taut in both flexion and extension. Volarly, there is a thick ligament, the volar (or palmar) plate that prevents hyperextension. The volar plates are composed of criss-crossing fibers that collapse and glide proximally during joint flexion and expand and move distally during joint extension.

The PIP joint has significant stability imparted by its bony anatomy, as the base of the middle phalanx has a prominent center that fits into a groove in the center of the proximal phalangeal

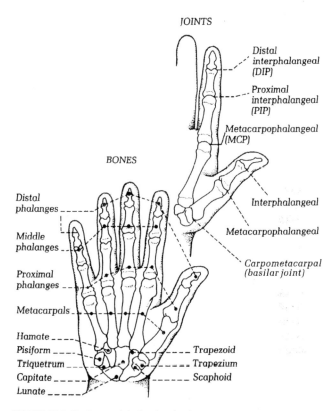

FIGURE 13-1 The bones of the hand and wrist.

head. The DIP joint has similar architecture. This bony configuration further stabilizes the interphalangeal joints against radial and ulnar deviation.

The MP joints of the fingers have a different osseous architecture than those of the interphalangeal joints (Fig. 13-2A and B). The metacarpal head is round and fits into the concavity of the proximal phalangeal base. This joint architecture is inherently less stable than that of the interphalangeal joints but allows radial and ulnar deviation of the MP joint when it is

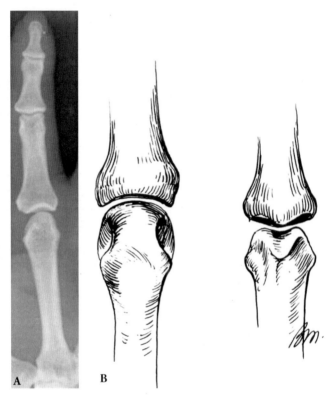

FIGURE 13-2 PA radiograph of a digit showing the difference in architecture between the DIP, PIP, and MP joints. The base of the middle phalanx has a prominent center that fits into a groove in the center of the proximal phalange's head. The DIP joint has a similar architecture. In comparison, the MP joint has a concave proximal phalangeal base articulating with a convex metacarpal head **(A)**. An X-ray of the finger MP and PIP joint osseous anatomy **(B)**. (Figure 13-2B from Rockwood & Green, 4th ed., Vol. 1, page 677, Fig. 11–75; with permission.).

extended. The MP joint also has collateral ligaments on either side and a volar plate to prevent hyperextension. However, the metacarpal head when viewed in the sagittal plane is cam shaped, causing the distance from the metacarpal head's center

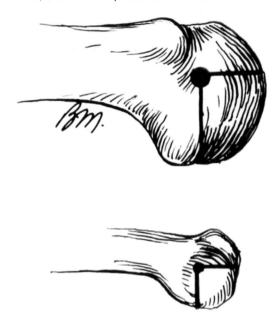

FIGURE 13-3 The metacarpal head is cam shaped, causing the distance from its center of rotation to its articular surface palmar to be longer than distal. The phalangeal head center of rotation on the other hand is more spherical and these two distances are equal. (Figure 13-3 from Rockwood and Green, 4th ed., Vol. 1, page 677, Fig. 11–76; with permission.).

of rotation to its articular surface to be longer in MP joint flexion than in extension (Fig. 13-3). Therefore, the MP joint's collateral ligaments are loose in extension and tight in flexion. This allows radioulnar deviation to occur in extension only, while providing increased stability in flexion, such as when grasping an object or making a fist.

Because of this cam effect, when the MP joint is splinted for any length of time, the collateral ligaments must be maintained in their lengthened position in flexion to prevent their shortening and contracture. Immobilization of the MP joint in extension will result in stiffness and a loss of flexion. Conversely, because the volar plates of the PIP and DIP joints have a tendency to scar and shorten, the interphalangeal joints are best immobilized in full extension. This optimal position of splinting, with the MP joint flexed and the PIP and DIP joints extended, is commonly referred to as the "intrinsic plus" position. Many commercial splints hold the fingers with the MP joints extended and the PIP and/or DIP joints flexed, a suboptimal position, which can lead to otherwise preventable stiffness and dysfunction.

THE THUMB

The thumb has only three articulations: the IP, MP, and trapeziometacarpal (TM) joints. The IP joint has architecture similar to the IP joints of the fingers and also functions as a hinge joint. The thumb MP joint is more complex than that of the fingers. While the MP joint of the thumb has a concave–convex architecture similar to that of the finger, the MP joint of the thumb has extremely strong ulnar and radial collateral ligaments that prevent radioulnar deviation in both flexion and extension. This facilitates pinch, where the thumb's MP joint has to provide stability in extension. This dependency on collateral ligaments for stability throughout motion explains why injury to these collateral ligaments is more disabling than the analogous injury to the fingers. The thumb's MP joint also has two sesamoid bones: one in each head of the flexor pollicis brevis that serve to increase the moment arm and in turn the flexor power of this muscle.

The thumb metacarpal joins the trapezium at the first carpometacarpal (CMC) joint or more precisely named the TM joint. The bony anatomy of the TM joint is a "double-saddle" joint, as the opposing surfaces of the thumb metacarpal and P1 resemble a horse's saddle. These opposing saddle-like surface face each other and are rotated perpendicular to each other. This highly specialized universal joint is responsible for most of the thumb's motion and allows for thumb opposition and pinch (Fig. 13-4). As the thumb opposes the fingers, it pronates, which facilitates pinching objects against the fingers.

The TM joint has little osseous stability and therefore relies on several ligaments for stability throughout its range of motion. An important ligament is the volar oblique (or "beak") ligament,

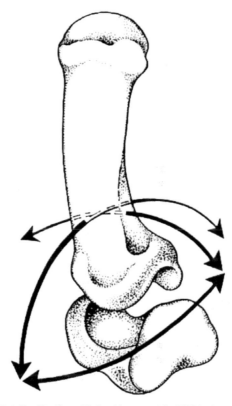

FIGURE 13-4 The "double-saddle" architecture of the TM joint between thumb metacarpal and trapezium.

which originates from the volar tubercle of the trapezium and attaches to the ulnar side of the proximal metacarpal "beak." Its main function is to prevent dorsal translation of the first metacarpal during pinch or grasp. Attenuation of the volar oblique ligament has been implicated in the pathogenesis of TM osteoarthritis. While this osseoligamentous arrangement provides for free mobility and adequate stability, it comes at the price of high contact forces, which may explain why the TM joint is the most commonly involved joint with arthritis in the hand.

THE WRIST

The carpus is composed of eight bones (Fig. 13-1): the scaphoid, lunate, triquetrum, pisiform, trapezium, trapezoid, capitate, and hamate organized into two rows: the proximal carpal row and the distal carpal row. The pisiform is essentially a sesamoid bone within the flexor carpi ulnaris tendon and is not part of the carpal row structure. It is surrounded by a soft tissue confluence. (Fig. 13-1 and Fig. 13-5)

The *distal carpal row* is composed of the trapezium, trapezoid, capitate, and hamate (Fig. 13-6). The trapezium has greater mobility, which allows it to move with the thumb. The remaining bones of the distal carpal row, however, are joined together by very strong ligaments that prevent substantial motion between them. The metacarpals are firmly anchored to the distal carpal row, especially along the index and middle finger rays. This stable central column facilitates power pinch. The ring and

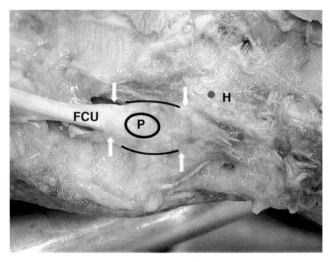

FIGURE 13-5 Pisiform and surrounding soft tissue confluence. Arrows point to a soft tissue confluence over the pisiform where its proximal pole gives attachment to the flexor carpi ulnaris tendon (FCU); P, pisiform; H, hamate. (Picture is courtesy of Ghazi Rayan MD).

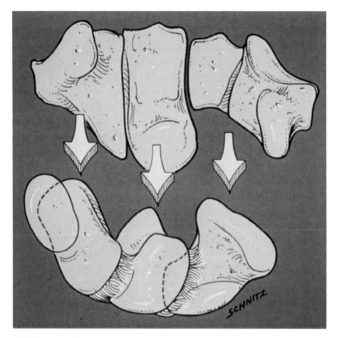

FIGURE 13-6 The carpal bones of the proximal (below) and distal (above) carpal rows.

small finger CMC joints have greater motion (and less stability) to allow the ulnar fingers to flex more and facilitate grasp. The small finger CMC joint allows 15–20° of flexion and the ring finger CMC joint allows 5–10° of flexion. Because of their articulations with the hamate, the fourth and fifth metacarpals supinate (rotate towards the thumb) during flexion to facilitate grasp and provide the ability to "cup" the hand.

The *proximal row* (Fig. 13-6) is composed of the scaphoid, lunate, and triquetrum. These have a very complex relationship with each other and the distal carpal row. In short, each of these bones is attached to the adjacent bones by ligaments, specifically the scapholunate interosseous ligament (SLIL) and the lunotriquetral interosseous ligament (LTIL), each named for the two bones they join. These two "intrinsic" ligaments (between carpal bones) cause the three bones of the proximal row to move together in unison with minimal motion allowed between them. However, the ligaments attaching the proximal carpal row to the distal carpal row on both sides of the wrist are weaker and allow motion between these two rows. In wrist flexion–extension, the proximal and distal carpal rows move together, into flexion and extension, respectively. However, the proximal carpal row also flexes in radial deviation and extends in ulnar deviation. The scaphoid bone serves as a link between the proximal and distal carpal rows, which predisposes it to being the most commonly fractured carpal bone.

It is noteworthy that no tendons insert into the carpal bones and that the carpal bones therefore move only in response to the tendon forces that insert distally into the hand. As the distal carpal row is firmly fixed to the metacarpal bases, where the wrist's tendons attach, the mobile proximal row functions as an intercalated (without direct control) segment during wrist motion. The complex carpal bone motions essentially allow wrist to replicate the motion of a ball and socket joint, such as the hip and shoulder.

In neutral deviation (i.e., midway between ulnar and radial deviation) the scaphoid and normally just over half (roughly 5/8) of the lunate articulate with the distal radius. This serves as the foundation of the radiocarpal articulation. The remainder of the lunate and the triquetrum articulate with the triangular fibrocartilage complex (TFCC) articular disk that is located just distal to the distal ulna and separates the ulnar head from the carpal bones. The TFCC is the major stabilizer of the distal radioulnar joint, that is, between the distal radius and ulna during forearm rotation.

The wrist is supported by strong volar ligaments between the distal radius and distal ulna and the carpus. These volar extrinsic ligaments provide the majority of radiocarpal stability and prevent ulnar translation of the wrist, whereby the carpal bones pathologically "slide down" the radial inclination of the distal radius so that greater than half of the lunate is no longer "covered" by the distal radius in neutral deviation. These ligaments are arranged in an inverted double-V pattern that allows flexion and extension of the proximal carpal row during radial and ulnar deviation, respectively.

The volar aspect of the lunocapitate articulation (the "Space of Poirier") is an area of weakness devoid of volar ligamentous support, which allows perilunate dislocations to occur.

The two dorsal ligaments of the wrist are thickenings in the dorsal joint capsule that provide secondary support to the wrist in maintaining carpal alignment. Both attach to the dorsal tubercle of the triquetrum, which forms the apex of a lateral V. The dorsal radiocarpal ligament attaches to the dorsal margin of the distal radius and has additional attachment to the LTIL to support that structure. The dorsal intercarpal ligament attaches to the trapezium and its fibers span the SLIL supporting its function.

History Taking and Examination of the Hand

Obtaining adequate history and conducting a thorough physical examination of the hand is crucial for accurate diagnosis and providing the appropriate treatment. This process should be tailored to specific conditions as will be discussed in each of the chapters later in this section. This chapter, however, is concerned with a review of the general clinical assessment of the hand that should be part of the specific evaluation for each system, such as peripheral nerves, vessels, tendons, bones, and joints.

TAKING A THOROUGH HISTORY

Taking history is both an art and science. Interviewing a patient has common elements among all specialties, but the way a question is phrased can elicit important information. With practice, interviewing a patient with a hand condition can be a focused and useful exercise.

With any patient an inquiry about the chief complaint is always the best way to begin. "What brings you here today?" is an open-ended question that commonly elicits most of the information you need for making a diagnosis. It is critical to let the patient take the time to finish the two to three sentences it usually takes to answer this question. This allows you to focus on the problem in your further history taking and examination.

Other key elements of the history are listed below:

Duration: How long the patient has had this condition and has it changed over time?

Mechanism: How did the injury/overuse occur, or what activity provokes pain? (work activities, sports, etc.)

Intensity: How painful is the problem, if it causes pain? Using a numeric scale of 0–10 can be helpful for monitoring the patient's pain over time.

Related complaints: Do other symptoms occur when the patient is having this particular complaint? Sometimes other sites of pain can be related.

Once you have these basic elements of the condition, other aspects of history taking include the following:

Past medical history: This is an inquiry about systemic diseases such as diabetes mellitus (which is a risk factor for trigger fingers and carpal tunnel syndrome), heart disease, gout, and inflammatory arthritic conditions such as rheumatoid disease. Additionally, it is important to ask about previous hand injuries or other hand disorders.

Past surgical history: Information should be obtained about any previous hand surgery, but any other surgery and complications related to those surgeries are important.

Medications: A complete list of both prescription and over-the-counter medications should be obtained. Patients on blood thinners (e.g., warfarin and dipyridamole) can have excessive bleeding at surgery or following injections. Certain herbal medications may interact with other pharmaceuticals; hence a record of these should be made as well.

Allergies: This includes allergies to medications, latex, tape, or environmental allergens.

Social history: Tobacco use is important to document because of its impact on bone and soft tissue healing. Alcohol abuse can have important implications for clotting mechanism and overall general health. Use of drugs and the last time they were taken are important information, particularly in the case of suspected drug abscess.

Family history and review of systems: The genetic component must be considered for congenital malformation and diseases such as Dupuytren's disease Ehler–Danlos and Madelung deformity.

Additionally, other issues may surface during the review of systems that may have an impact on the chief complaint.

PHYSICAL EXAMINATION
Inspection

During physical examination of the hand, it is optimal to be seated across from the patient and to have their hands resting on a table of comfortable height for both parties. Knowledge of the surface anatomy of the hand (Fig. 14-1) is the key in assessing the hand

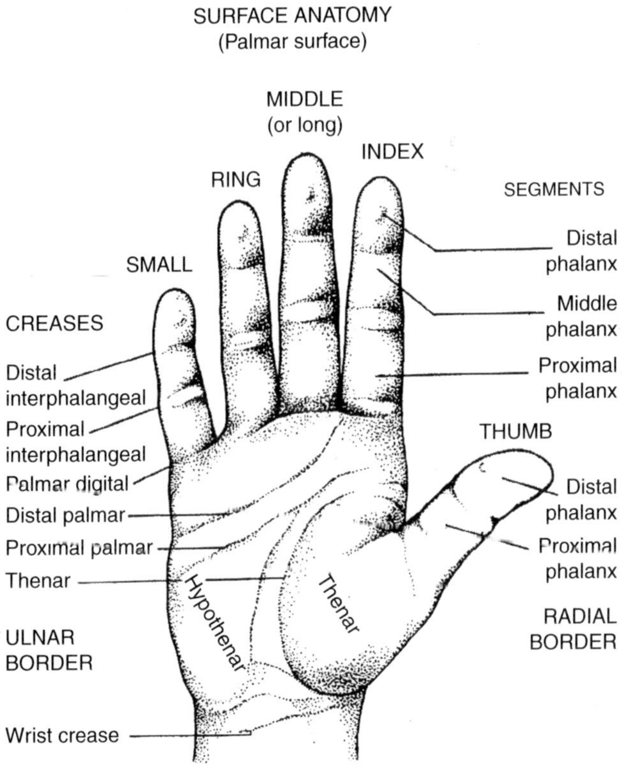

SURFACE ANATOMY
(Palmar surface)

FIGURE 14-1 Surface anatomy of the hand.

and its varied joints. Examination begins with inspection of the hands to look for swelling, masses, or deformities. Scars from previous surgery or injury should be observed as well as amputations and nail deformities. By inspecting both hands simultaneously, one can compare them side-by-side which will reveal any asymmetry.

Palpation

Syndesmotic system: A goniometer can be used to measure the range of motion (ROM) of various joints of the upper extremity (Table 14-1 and Fig. 14-2).

Osseous system: The shafts of the radius and ulna should be palpated along their lengths, and the distal radius and ulna are considered separately. The radiocarpal joint is palpated dorsally, noting any masses or tenderness. The distal radioulnar joint is evaluated, noting any tenderness. The examiner's finger is placed at the

TABLE 14-1	Range of Motion Testing		
Anatomic region	**Extension**	**Flexion**	**Other ROM**
Shoulder	40–60°	180° (forward flexion/ elevation	Abduction 120° Adduction 50° Internal/external rotation 90°
Elbow	0°	130–140°	
Forearm			Pronation/supination each 90° from neutral (thumb up)
Wrist	30–70°	40–80°	Radial deviation, 10–30° Ulnar deviation, 20–40°
MCP	0°	90°	
PIP	0°	120°	
DIP	0°	40–50°	

Normal

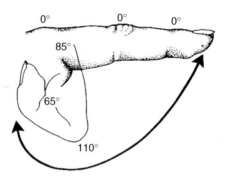

FIGURE 14-2 ROM of digital joints.

ulnocarpal sulcus, and the ulnar "fovea" is palpated, just distal to the ulnar styloid.

The midcarpal joint is palpated, followed by the metacarpal bases and moving up to the shafts of the metacarpals. Next the metacarpophalangeal (MP), proximal interphalangeal (PIP), and distal interphalangeal (DIP) joints are examined for tenderness or instability.

The basal joint of the thumb is assessed by feeling for the depression between the base of the first metacarpal and the trapezium. Just proximally, the examiner may palpate the scapho—trapezio–trapezoid joint for tenderness.

Neurologic system: This includes motor and sensory evaluation of the median, radial, and ulnar nerves.

Special Tests

There are many *special tests* that should be used while examining the hand. The most common will be discussed.

Compression Neuropathy
Carpal Tunnel Syndrome
• Phalen test is classically performed by asking the patient to flex their elbows and wrists to 90° for one minute and noting whether

TABLE 14-2	Motor/Sensory Nerve Examination in the Hand	

Peripheral nerve	Sensory distribution	Motor testing/ function
Median	Volar surface of thumb, index, and middle fingers	FDS = digital PIP flexion FDP index/middle = digital DIP flexion index / middle Thenar muscles = thumb opposition
Radial	Radial dorsal half of the hand Dorsum of the first web space	EPL = thumb IP joint extension EDC = extension of MP joints of all fingers
Ulnar	Volar small finger and ulnar half of the ring finger	Lumbrical muscles = flex MP and extend PIP joints Intrinsic muscles = digital adduction and abduction

this reproduces the symptoms of numbness and tingling in the median nerve distribution: the thumb, index, middle, and radial half of the ring finger (Fig. 14-3).

- Tinel test is performed by tapping over the median nerve at the wrist (in line with the middle finger) and noting whether this causes electrical shock-like sensations along the nerve distribution (Fig. 14-4).
- Durkan carpal tunnel compression test is performed by compressing the median nerve at the wrist with two of the examiner's fingers and noting whether this reproduces the symptoms of numbness and tingling.

Cubital Tunnel Syndrome. It is caused by compression of the ulnar nerve at the cubital tunnel or medial elbow. The patient's complains are numbness in the small finger and the ulnar half of the ring along with weakness of the hand. The patient will have positive Tinel sign at the retro-condylar groove.

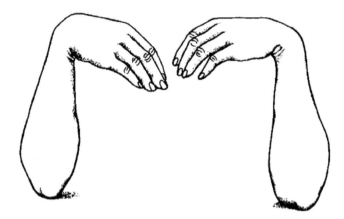

FIGURE 14-3 Phalen test.

- The elbow flexion test is performed by asking the patient to flex their elbow maximally for 1 minute. This provokes numbness in the ulnar digits.

Thoracic Outlet Syndrome. It is due to compression of the subclavian vessels and brachial plexus, especially the lower trunk in the cervico–thoraco–brachial region. This can cause paresthesias and pain but is considered a clinical diagnosis. Sometimes the condition is caused by a cervical rib.

- *Roos overhead test*: This provocative test is performed by asking the patient to hold the elbows fully extended and shoulders fully abducted overhead while repeatedly making and opening fists on both hands. A positive test will reproduce paresthesias and or hand pallor.
- *Hyperabduction test*: The shoulder is fully extended and abducted, which may diminish the pulse and will provoke hand paresthesias.
- *Adson and costoclavicular tests*: These are done by turning the patient's head toward the symptomatic side while tilting and extending the neck away from the painful arm or by assuming the exaggerated military maneuver of retracting the shoulders. The patient then inhales deeply, and the physician palpates for diminish or loss of radial pulse. The patient is asked to breath normally while inquiring about paresthesias on the symptomatic arm.

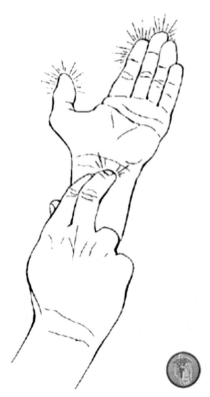

FIGURE 14-4 Tinel test.

Tendinopathies

Lateral Elbow Tendinopathy

- Commonly known as tennis elbow. The patient has tenderness directly at or just distal to the lateral epicondyle.
- Resistive wrist and middle finger extension and resistive forearm supination while the elbow extended provokes pain in the lateral elbow.

DeQuervain Tenosynovitis

- More commonly seen in women. It is an inflammatory tenosynovitis of the extensor pollicis brevis and abductor of the thumb

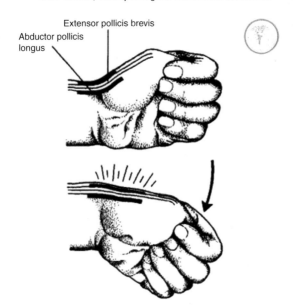

Abductor pollicis longus

Extensor pollicis brevis

FIGURE 14-5 Finkelstein test.

in the first dorsal extensor compartment and characterized by pain and tenderness at the dorsal radial wrist
- Finkelstein maneuver is performed by asking the patient to place their thumb inside their closed fist and then passively ulnar deviating the wrist (Fig. 14-5). Another method is to passively adduct the patient's thumb. A positive test occurs when this provokes severe pain.

Trigger Finger/Thumb

The patient is asked to demonstrate clicking or locking that is perceived at the PIP joint of the finger [or interphalangeal (IP) joint of the thumb], although the pathology is at the A-1 pulley which is located over the MP joint, just distal to the distal palmar crease. There is also tenderness at the volar base of the finger at the A-1 pulley area.

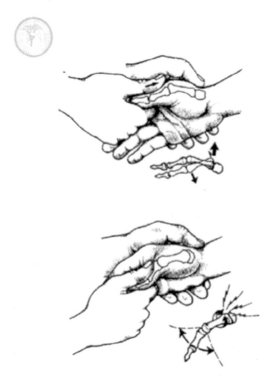

FIGURE 14-6 Grind test.

Arthritis

Trapeziometacarpal (Basilar Thumb) Joint Arthritis

- *Grind test*: This is done by grasping the thumb metacarpal shaft and by applying an axial load to the trapeziometacarpal joint (Fig. 14-6). A positive test provokes pain and gives the sensation of the cartilage surfaces roughly grinding together or crepitance occurring.

Another test is simple palpation of the trapeziometacarpal by sliding the examiner's finger proximally along the radial and volar aspect of the first metacarpal and dropping into the palpable ridge between the metacarpal base and the trapezium. This provokes pain in the arthritic joint.

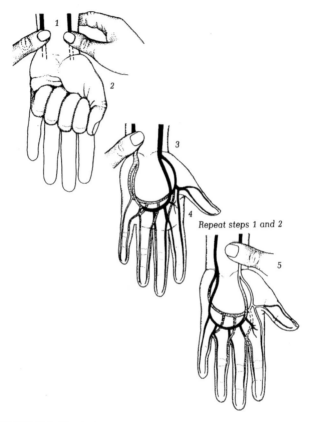

FIGURE 14-7 Allen test.

Vascular Occlusive Disease

Thrombosis of Ulnar or Digital Arteries

- *Allen test:* This is performed by having the patient flex and extend the digits multiple times, that is, making fists while the examiner occludes the radial and ulnar arteries at the wrist. Digital flexion moves blood out of the hand and the pallor will be manifest. The examiner then releases pressure over one artery. The same is performed for the second artery. Normally there should be blood flow and return of color to the hand in 2–5 seconds (Fig. 14-7). Lack of flow through one of the arteries constitute a positive test.

CHAPTER 15

Peronychium

Examination of the perionychium begins with the inspection of the nail plate and its surrounding soft tissue structures. Nail abnormality or subtle deformity becomes apparent when compared to adjacent normal nail. Range of motion is assessed by asking the patient to flex and extend the distal interphalangeal joint while the examiner holds the proximal interphalangeal joint extended. Stability of the distal interphalangeal joint should be assessed to rule out associated ligament attenuation or rupture. The extensor digitorum communis and flexor digitorum profundus tendon function also should be evaluated to rule out their injury. Palpation of the fingertip will detect areas of tenderness or swelling, stability of the nail plate, and distal phalanx. Vascular sufficiency is assessed by capillary refill testing. This is done both on the skin of the pulp and at the nail plate by pressing these areas and observing for blanching followed by brisk return of circulation. Light touch sensibility is evaluated on the volar, radial and ulnar sides of the fingertip. Open wounds should be visually inspected after cleaning any blood clots.

A normal nail plate is smooth and shiny, with a visible lunula proximally. The plate should be adherent to the underlying nail matrix without instability or mobility. Trauma to the nail can present as a fractured nail plate and open nail bed laceration, or as a closed subungual hematoma. Nail damage and subungual hematoma must raise the suspicion of a fracture of the distal phalanx; hence radiographs of the finger should be obtained. If the nail plate is damaged, this implies sterile matrix injury, which may require surgical repair. If the hard nail plate is unstable, this usually requires replacement in the nail socket under the nail fold with or without anchoring sutures to protect the underlying germinal and sterile matrix.

A subungual hematoma most commonly occurs after a crushing injury to the digit. This may be associated with an intact or

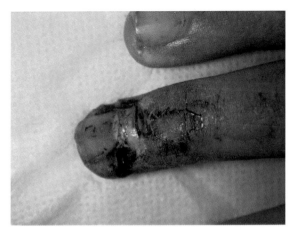

FIGURE 15-1 A subungual hematoma is associated with laceration to the nail matrix especially when proximal nail avulsion is present. (Picture is courtesy of Ghazi Rayan MD).

partially intact nail plate and underlying blood accumulation. Because of the limited space beneath the nail, a subungual hematoma can exert pressure on the sensitive nailbed and be quite painful. Evacuation of a small subungual hematoma by placing holes in the nail plate can relieve pain; however, large subungual hematomas require removal of the nail plate and exploration for possible repair (Fig. 15-1). Failure to restore nail matrix anatomy after lacerations will result in nail deformity (Fig. 15-2).

Remote trauma to the nail matrix can cause nail deformities. Ridging of the nail can occur after damage to the sterile nail matrix with residual scarring. If the germinal matrix, which produces most of the nail plate, is damaged, a portion or the entire nail may not grow.

Tumors and masses of the nail unit can present in varied ways. A glomus tumor, originating from the neuro-arterial apparatus or glomus body, can cause a bluish discoloration under the nail and pain particularly with temperature change, that is, cold hypersensitivity. Surgical removal of the glomus tumor will generally relieve the patient's symptoms. Mucous cysts or other masses situated at the proximal nail fold and the germinal matrix can cause ridging of the nail due to pressure on the cells (Fig. 15-3A and B). Tumors involving

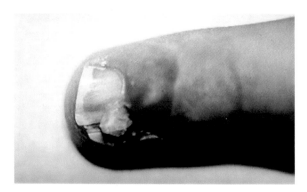

FIGURE 15-2 Nail deformity following unrepaired nail matrix laceration. (Picture is courtesy of Ghazi Rayan MD).

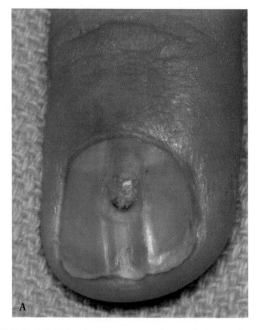

FIGURE 15-3 Nail ridging due to pressure on the germinal matrix from a mass (**A**) (Picture is courtesy of Jennifer Wolf MD) and mucous cyst (**B**). (*continued*)

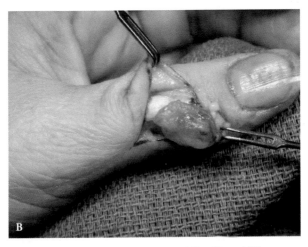

FIGURE 15-3 (*Continued*) (Picture is courtesy of Ghazi Rayan MD).

melanocytes, including benign nevi and malignant melanoma, can cause dark pigmented lines under the nail due to transport of abnormal cells initially located on the germinal matrix. Metastases of primary malignant tumors to the distal phalanx are rare but can cause nail deformity or erosion through the nail bed.

Infection of the perionychium has multiple clinical presentations. Infection of the nail pad or hyponychium and subcutaneous tissue of the pulp is known as a felon. The pulp becomes erythematous, swollen, and quite tender. Felons require surgical drainage by releasing the numerous small vertical fibrous bands and decompression of adipose compartments. Paronychia is an infection of the paronychium, which presents with swelling and pain at the lateral nail fold, sometimes with drainage of purulent fluid. This can be exquisitely painful due to the pressure from the collected pus. Surgical drainage requires removing the adjacent portion of the nail plate and drainage of any purulence under the paronychium (Fig. 15-4). Herpetic whitlow is a viral infection of the perionychium, which is commonly encountered among healthcare workers. The patient presents with intense burning pain, swelling, erythema, and characteristic small clear fluid-filled vesicles. Herpetic whitlow has a chronic course and its treatment should be palliative local care. Surgery is contraindicated as it may be complicated by dissemination and viral meningitis.

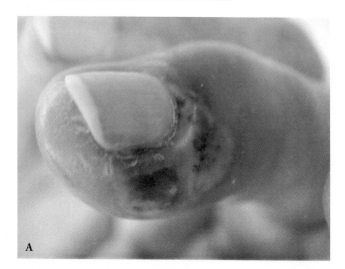

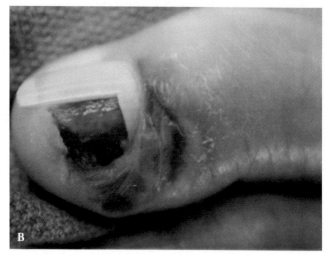

FIGURE 15-4 A paronychia or bacterial infection of the lateral nail fold (**A**) and following excision of portion of the nail plate and drainage of a large abscess (**B**). (Picture is courtesy of Ghazi Rayan MD).

CHAPTER 16

Skin

EXAMINATION

Examination of the skin of the hand begins with a general inspection followed by a detailed palpation of areas of interest. This evaluation is facilitated by adequate lighting and, when indicated, by the use of magnification and/or a Woods lamp. Gloves should be worn if the patient has open wounds or obvious lesions or complains of itching. During the examination, particular attention should be directed toward evaluation of the following:

Color: The dorsal skin should be flesh-toned appropriate for the race of the patient.

Temperature and Turgor: The back of the hand should be used to assess skin temperature for excessive warmth or coolness. Turgor may be assessed by pinching the skin between the examiners thumb and index finger for a few seconds. Normally hydrated skin will recoil when released while dehydrated skin will remain tented. However, when interpreting this test it must be kept in mind that elderly patients' skin will often tent, particularly over the dorsum of the hand, even with adequate hydration. In addition to dehydration, skin elasticity can be altered by other pathologic conditions such as Ehlers Danlos syndrome (excessive laxity) or scleroderma (excessive tightness).

Moisture: Dry skin presenting as flaking and cracked can be caused by the use of irritating soaps, exposure to industrial solvents, excessive solar exposure, or diseases such as hypothyroidism. Like tenting skin with a pinch test, dryness may also be age related, being more common in the elderly.

Scars: The cause should be determined if possible including the date of injury or surgery. Often observation of and query as to the cause will elicit a history of surgery that the patient has not previously mentioned.

Masses and lesions: Location, size, and color of masses or lesions should be accurately recorded along with the date they were first noted by the patient. Light palpation of the mass or lesion is then carried out to help determine depth, mobility, consistency, and degree of tenderness.

Birthmarks/moles: These lesions require special attention. Location, color, shape, and size need to be accurately documented and consideration should be given to entering a photographic image with a metric indicator in the medical record for future reference. The ABCD's of melanoma detection, a potentially fatal malignant skin lesion, should be accurately assessed and documented:

- A = asymmetry: one half is different from the other half.
- B = border irregularity: the edges are notched, uneven, or blurred.
- C = color: the color is uneven with shades of black, brown, and tan present simultaneously.
- D = diameter: greater than 6 mm (the size of a standard pencil eraser).

DISCRIPTIVE TERMS

Like all branches of medicine there is a specific language associated with the description of dermatologic lesions. Accurate use of these terms greatly facilitates interspecialty communication and helps keep the medical record consistent throughout its chronology. Common terms utilized to describe frequently encountered primary skin lesions are as follows:

Macule: A flat, small (1 cm or less), colored lesion such as encountered in measles. These lesions are by definition visible but not palpable.

Papule: An elevated, sharply circumscribed, small (1 cm or less) lesion that may or may not be pigmented. Common papular lesions are warts, nevi, or Molluscum contagiosum.

Nodules: Papules greater than 1 cm in diameter. Nodules may be visibly raised above the surrounding skin or palpable within the skin.

Vesicles (small blisters): Fluid-filled lesions under 1 cm in diameter which can be seen in a variety of viral infections such as Herpes simplex or chickenpox.

Bullae (large blisters): Fluid-filled lesions 1 cm or greater in diameter as encountered in second-degree burns, fractures, and insect bite reactions.

Pustules: Elevated, sharply circumscribed lesions, less than 1 cm in diameter that are filled with pus. On occasion these infections may affect hair follicles resulting in a condition termed *folliculitis*.

Cysts: Walled-off lesions containing fluid or semisolid material. Examples include pilar and epidermoid inclusion cysts.

Wheals: Raised flesh-colored or erythematous evanescent lesion. Wheals generally last less than 24 hours, during which time they may change in shape and size. Wheals are commonly seen in allergic drug reactions known as "hives."

Primary lesions should be distinguished from secondary lesions, which result from alteration, usually traumatic, to the primary lesion. Examples are excoriation and ulceration from scratching of primary lesions, or crusts of dried blood, serum, scales, and pus that are the end result of diseases such as infectious dermatitis or more advanced skin cancer.

COMMON CLINICAL CONDITIONS

Congenital skin conditions of the hand can be isolated lesions, associated with other congenital anomalies, or the result of a generalized skin condition.

Syndactyly is the most common congenital condition of the hand and can involve skin alone, underlying bony structures, and on occasion can be associated with other congenital anomalies. Simple syndactyly is isolated to the skin and occurs when the normal processes of digital separation and web space formation fails to a variable degree. This simple form results in fusion of adjacent digits with a web that may extend to the fingertip, *complete syndactyly*, or be *incomplete* where the web ends somewhere distant to the point of the normal commissure. While any web space may be affected the most common fusion is between the ring and the long finger. Treatment consists of surgical separation of the involved digits, reconstruction of an appropriate web, and skin grafting of any areas of skin deficiency.

Other congenital lesions, which may be encountered in the hand, include isolated congenital pigmented nevus and digital fibroma of infancy. In addition patients may present with hand involvement from generalized skin disorders such as Ehlers–Danlos syndrome or epidermolysis bullosa.

Congenital nevi may be small and require no treatment other than observation, or may present as giant melanocytic nevi that are not only disfiguring but also carry some malignant potential. Treatment of large melanocytic nevi may require multiple-staged surgeries with complex reconstruction to preserve function of the involved hand.

Digital fibroma of infancy is a benign but aggressive lesion which is confined to the digits. Over 80% of the cases arise before one year of age and appears early as a small dome-shaped painless mass near the interphalangeal joint. With time these lesions may regress or become rapidly expansile requiring excision and even in some cases amputation.

Ehlers–Danlos syndrome and epidermolysis bullosa are both hereditary disorders that affect the entire skin envelope. In Ehlers–Danlos syndrome the skin of the dorsum of the hand is hyperextensible. This laxity itself requires no treatment but the skin may be thin and more vulnerable to injury than normal integument. In contrast, epidermolysis bullosa is a severe blistering disorder of the skin which leads to progressive pseudosyndactyly (referred to as epidermal cocoons) as well as flexion contractures of the digits both of which frequently require surgical management. The aim of surgery in these children is the establishment and maintenance of independent digits that are capable of flexion and extension. This requires a combination of release of the cocoons followed by splinting and contracture release with skin grafting.

Trauma to the skin of the hand may be encountered as isolated lacerations, avulsions, as a component of crush injuries, as well as burns from heat, cold, or chemicals. Treatment needs to be individualized based on the mechanism, cleanliness of the wound, time which has elapsed since injury, and other associated injuries.

Infections of the skin of the hand are usually associated with trauma with inoculation of micro-organisms or chronic exposure to irritants that lead to breakdown of normal protective mechanisms. These may present as localized infections confined to anatomical areas, such as the pulp and web spaces, or present as a more generalized cellulitis with or without cutaneous lymphatic involvement.

Treatment consists of drainage of any localized purulent collections and systemic antibiotics.

A variety of benign and malignant skin tumors occur in the hand. Benign tumors include sebaceous cysts, cutaneous horns, common warts, pyogenic granuloma, keratoacanthoma, dermatofibroma, and a variety of pigmented nevi. Pyogenic granulomas are tumorous growths often attributed to prior trauma but whose precise etiology remains unknown. They appear as reddish nodules on the skin that when traumatized demonstrate a tendency for profuse bleeding. Initial treatment of these lesions consists of repeated applications of silver nitrate, but if this fails to control the lesion then surgical excision will be required.

Keratoacanthomas are rapidly growing skin tumors that characteristically contain a central keratin plug. While spontaneous regression may occur these lesions are very difficult to differentiate clinically and histologically from squamous cell carcinomas (SCC); hence complete excision is recommended.

Common malignant skin tumors include squamous cell carcinomas, basal cell carcinomas (BCC), and malignant melanoma. SCC of the dorsum of the hand is unique in that it occurs at a higher incidence in this location than the less aggressive BCC. Both types of tumor are treated by excision and both are often related to sun exposure. SCC may appear as a slow growing wart-like lesion beneath, near, or under the fingernail, or as large ulcerated or exophytic tumor. With SCC less than 2 cm in diameter, 4 mm of surgical margin excision is adequate. With lesions greater than 2 cm this margin should be expanded to 6 mm. Full-thickness skin excision is recommended including some subcutaneous fat. With distal finger lesions, fingertip amputation may be required.

BCC like SCC may have a variety of appearances and may present as areas of skin atrophy, pink to reddish discoloration, pigmented lesions that may be confused with melanoma, elevated pearly nodules, or ulcerated lesions. Successful treatment of BCC may be achieved by a variety of techniques, including electro-dissection and curettage, freezing, chemical application, as well as conventional excision. Recommended margins for BCC are 4 mm for lesions less than 2 cm in diameter and larger margins or Mohs micrographic surgery for lesions greater than 2 cm in diameter and those that display histologically aggressive features.

Malignant melanoma is an aggressive cutaneous malignancy of increasing frequency that has a higher potential for metastasis with increased depth of invasion. In its least aggressive form it is confined to the epidermis and is referred to as lentigo maligna or melanoma in situ. This type lesion has little or no metastatic potential. Other more serious presentations are described based on clinical appearance and include superficial spreading melanoma (the most common form), nodular melanoma, and acral lentiginous melanoma, which is a variant found on the palmar surface. Depth of invasion of these lesions is graded histologically by the Breslow level system which is predictive of metastatic potential. Grading determines how aggressive surgery needs to be and whether sampling of regional lymph nodes by sentinel node biopsy is required. A notable exception to this is in the case of subungual melanoma where the involved tissue is of compressed nature and the Breslow system may not be accurate. In this instance sentinel node biopsy is always recommended and amputation is indicated, usually at the distal interphalangeal joint level.

SURGICAL RELEVANCE

While almost all surgery involves gaining access through the skin, primary surgery of the skin itself is indicated in trauma, and treatment of masses and select lesions. Surgery in these instances may consist of simple immediate or delayed wound closure supplemented, when necessary with some mobilization of adjacent tissue by undermining (Fig. 16-1). Alternatively, in the face of traumatic soft tissue loss, surgery may require complex reconstructive techniques such as the use of skin grafts or flaps. These reconstructive techniques may also be useful in providing soft tissue coverage after debridement and stabilization of complex open fractures, in the treatment of osteomyelitis, or after major ablative procedures.

Simple excisions can be performed using local anesthesia alone or in conjunction with mild sedation. To provide localized anesthesia, the anesthetic (most commonly lidocaine and/or marcaine) is injected around the operative site. For cutaneous injection a small bore needle such as a 25 or 30 gauge should be used to minimize patient discomfort. Alternatively, regional nerve blocks may be used for many minor upper extremity and hand procedures.

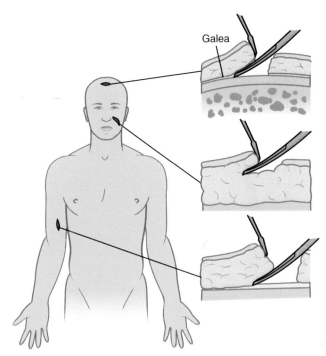

Galea

FIGURE 16-1 Schematic drawing demonstrating the various levels of under-mining that can be done based on anatomical site and depth of subcutaneous tissue.

Most simple skin excisions can be closed in one layer; however, two-layer closure including subcutaneous tissue is appropriate if excessive tension exists. Skin repair is done by a variety of suture patterns (Fig. 16-2).

Skin grafting is indicated when the wound cannot be closed primarily without excessive tension and following release of congenital or acquired contractures where a skin deficiency is present. Skin grafts may be either split or full-thickness graft (Fig. 16-3). Split-thickness grafts contain varying thicknesses of dermis while a full-thickness grafts contains the entire dermis as well as adnexal structures such as sweat glands, sebaceous glands, hair follicles, and capillaries. Because

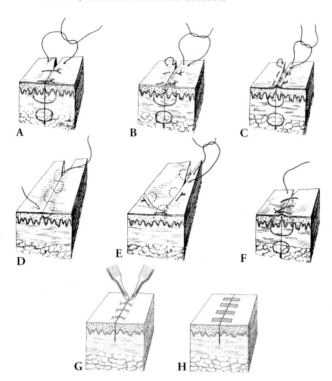

FIGURE 16-2 Possible suture patterns in skin closure. **A:** Simple interrupted. **B:** Vertical mattress. **C:** Horizontal mattress. **D:** Subcuticular continuous. **E:** Half-buried horizontal mattress. **F:** Continuous over-and-over. **G:** Staples. **H:** Skin tapes.

these two different type grafts vary in the quantity of dermis present they also vary in the degree of primary and secondary contracture.

Primary contracture is the immediate recoil demonstrated by a newly harvested graft as a result of the elastin present in the dermis. The more dermis the graft has the more primary contracture will occur. Secondary contracture occurs once the graft is placed on to its recipient bed. This scar contracture reduces both the size of the graft and the interface with its recipient bed and the circumference of the area. The propensity for secondary contracture is greater in split-thickness graft where less dermis is present than full-thickness grafts. In general, the

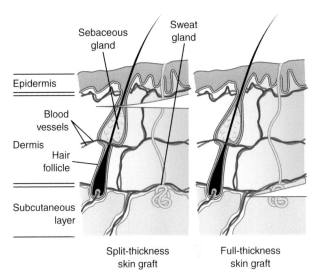

FIGURE 16-3 Skin grafts are divided into two main types: split-thickness skin grafts and full-thickness skin grafts.

thinner the skin graft the greater the secondary contracture; however, the nature of the graft is not the sole determinant of secondary contracture. The graft bed plays a role with a graft, placed directly on to fascia or a fresh tangentially excised wound, contracting less than those placed onto granulation tissue. The severity of secondary contracture is also greater among pediatric patients than adults.

Split-thickness skin grafts are most commonly harvested from the upper thigh or even higher by positioning the donor site over the muscle belly of the tensor fascia lata to allow for coverage of the donor site with clothing. Alternatively, grafts may be harvested from the inner aspect of the upper arm. The harvest of the graft may be performed with a hand-held knife; but frequently it is taken with an air or electric-powered instrument called a dermatome, which can harvest grafts of various thicknesses (Fig. 16-4).

Full-thickness skin grafts are commonly used in hand surgery and contain epidermis and full-thickness dermis. These types of grafts vary in thickness based on the location of the donor site. Common sites for full-thickness skin graft harvest for hand surgery

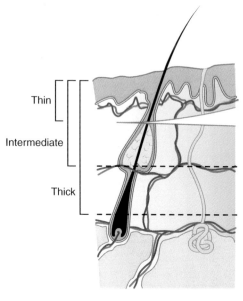

Split-thickness
skin graft

FIGURE 16-4 Depiction of the various thicknesses of split-thickness skin graft may be harvested by adjusting the setting of the dermatome.

are the hypothenar border of the hand, the volar wrist crease, the medial arm, and the groin crease. Glabrous donor sites are usually preferred. While full-thickness skin grafts undergo more primary contracture they offer the advantages of less secondary scar contracture than split-thickness skin grafts; and in many situations they result in less donor morbidity/scarring, provide a better color match, and result in less contour defect at the recipient site.

Skin graft "take" depends on the ability of the graft to obtain nutrients and vascular in-growth from the recipient bed. This process occurs in three phases. The first phase occurs between 24 and 48 hours and consists of direct absorption of nutrients from the recipient bed by a process referred to as *plasmatic imbibition*. The second phase is called *inosculation* and is initiated when the recipient and donor end capillaries align, resulting in the formation of direct anastomoses. In the third phase there is in-growth of new capillaries into the graft in a process appropriately called *revascularization*.

More complex reconstructive techniques include the use of skin flaps. Unlike a graft, flaps have their own blood supply. Flaps are indicated when the recipient bed would not support a graft, when further operations are planned in the wound site, for improved contour or function, and when immediate coverage is required for exposed vital structures (tendons, nerves, and blood vessels) and/or orthopedic hardware. Flaps can be developed locally, regionally, or be transferred to the defect site from remote anatomical sites by staged transfer or microsurgical techniques.

Flaps developed locally are moved into the defect site by advancement, rotation, or transposition (Fig. 16-5). These flaps may

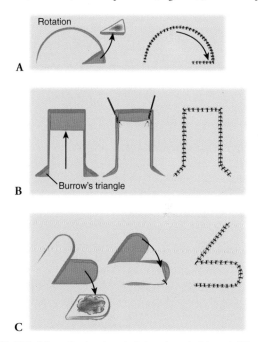

FIGURE 16-5 Schematic drawing depicting the principles of (**A**) rotation, (**B**) advancement, and (**C**) transposition flaps.

be axial and incorporate a known vascular supply or be random such that they are dependent on dermal plexuses.

Regional flaps usually are transferred as direct axial pattern flaps based on a named artery for their supply. Examples of this flap that can be used for hand coverage are the first dorsal metacarpal artery flap (Fig. 16-6A–C), posterior interosseous artery flap, and the radial forearm flap. Distant flaps have the advantage that they can bring in like tissue from a distant site in the

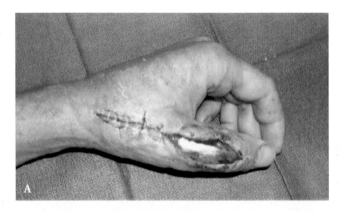

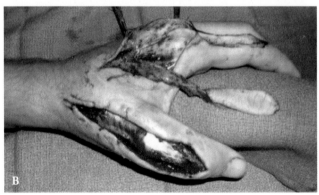

FIGURE 16-6 A: Degloving injury to the thumb. **B:** First dorsal metacarpal artery flap. (*continued*)

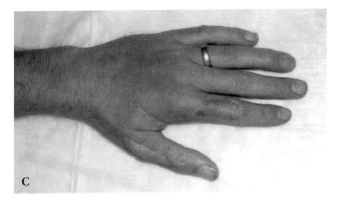

FIGURE 16-6 (*Continued*) **C:** Postoperatively. (Picture is courtesy of Ghazi Rayan MD).

face of an otherwise devastating injury. The flaps are moved by staged transfer or microsurgical techniques that allow for immediate revascularization and the potential for functional reinnervation.

Staged transfer is most commonly used in the upper extremity to transfer a groin flap based on the superficial circumflex iliac artery (Fig. 16-7A–C).

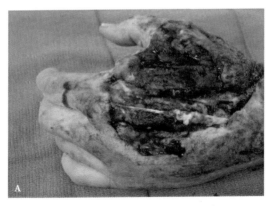

FIGURE 16-7 A: Degloving injury of the hand. (*continued*)

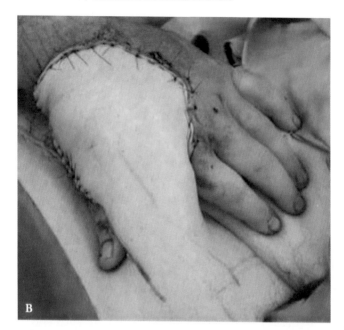

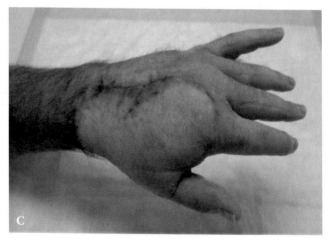

FIGURE 16-7 (*Continued*) **B:** Groin flap. **C:** Postoperatively. (Picture is courtesy of Ghazi Rayan MD).

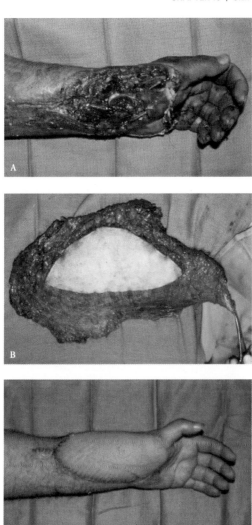

FIGURE 16-8 A: Degloving injury to the forearm. **B:** Free latissimus dorsi flap. **C:** Postoperatively. (Picture is courtesy of Steve Peterson MD).

Alternatively, distant tissue consisting of muscle, fascia, bone, or combinations of these three tissues is dissected free of its donor site based on its major arterial supply and then revascularized at the recipient site by microsurgical reconstruction of both arterial in-flow and venous outflow. An example is the latissimus dorsi flap that is based on the thoracodorsal artery (Fig. 16-8A–C). When indicated the dominant nerve supply may also be moved with the flap and connected to a recipient nerve to supply sensation to the flap and/or functional re-innervation such that muscle contraction is possible within the flap.

CHAPTER 17

Subcutaneous Tissue

EXAMINATION

Clinical examination of the subcutaneous tissue in the hand and fingers is important for evaluating lacerations and subcutaneous disorders such as masses and infections. The examination must include inspection and palpation.

Inspection for lacerations should assess their length and proximity to tendinous and neurovascular structures. Posture of a digit may give a clue to associated tendon injuries. Masses are to be inspected for their size, shape, and location and for any changes in the overlying skin. In case of infections, erythema, diffuse swelling, draining sinuses, or necrosis may be observed.

Palpation for laceration may include the presence of foreign bodies such as glass or gravel after administering local anesthetic. Hypoesthesia and anesthesia should be assessed prior to administering anesthetic. Loss of sensory function is encountered with associated peripheral nerve injuries (see nerve Chapter 21).

For masses palpation will differentiate between solid tumors or neoplasms and tumor-like conditions or cystic lesions. The latter diagnosis is confirmed by a fluctuation consistency and by transillumination (Fig. 17-1A and B). Palpation for tenderness will confirm the painful nature of these lesions and its level of intensity. In case of infection, palpation will be associated with excruciating pain accompanied by increased skin temperature. Decreased skin temperature is encountered in ischemic hands and digits and in vasospastic conditions (see Chapter 8).

CLINICAL CONDITIONS AND TREATMENT

Superficial lacerations are caused by sharp objects such as a knife, glass, or metal. Lacerations of the palm superficial to the deep

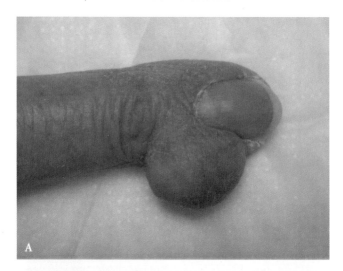

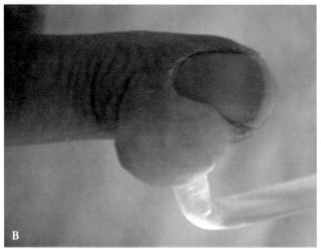

FIGURE 17-1 A ganglion cyst from the distal interphalangeal joint (**A**) that transilluminated against the light (**B**). (Picture courtesy of Ghazi Rayan MD).

fascia are unlikely to affect the tendons or neurovascular structures, but the examiner must confirm their lack of involvement. This is best done by first assessing digital motion, vascularity, and sensation and then examining the wound under local anesthesia. Similarly when examining the dorsum of the hand and fingers there is a higher likelihood that an innocuous appearing wound may hide an injury to a deeper important structure such as tendons.

Fingertip amputations are a common problem for the hand surgeon. Treatment varies based on the anatomy and direction of the amputation. The treatment objective is to maintain length, retain sensibility, and provide painless well-padded fingertip. The surgeon should balance the maintenance of digital length with a tension-free well-padded closure that can provide a painless digital pulp for pinch and fine motor skills. The wound is examined for the presence of exposed bone in planning the appropriate treatment of the fingertip injury. Radiographs allow confirmation of an associated bony loss or fracture. In addition, nail bed repair may be necessary depending on the level of amputation (see Chapter 15 for additional details regarding the perionychium).

Treatment options are largely determined by the location and geometry of the skin and soft tissue loss. Primary closure is an option if minimal tissue loss is present, although a tension-free closure is imperative. A smaller wound, classically described as 1×1 cm, without exposed bone may be allowed to heal by secondary intention. This can be an excellent option that often provides near normal aesthetics and sensation. A somewhat larger defect may be allowed to heal by secondary intention in the pediatric patient. Full-thickness skin grafting for distal tip amputations with skin or pulp loss is limited by inadequate padding of the pulp, diminished sensory function, and potential for cold sensitivity.

When the bone is exposed, shortening and primary closure may be performed in the fingers but length should be maintained whenever possible, especially in the thumb. A volar V-Y advancement flap (Fig. 17-2) provides an excellent closure in most patients except for those with a volar oblique injury. In those patients, lateral V-Y flaps can be utilized although the skin is less mobile. There are a variety of additional, staged flaps described for fingertip closure that allow maintenance of length and sensibility including cross-finger flap and thenar flap (Fig. 17-3). A Moberg flap may be

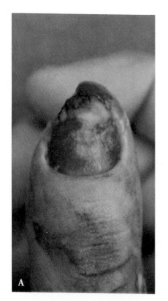

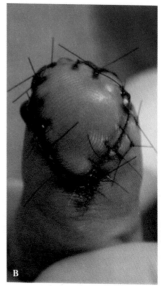

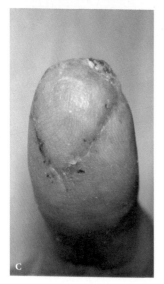

FIGURE 17-2 A–C: V-Y lap coverage for thumb tip amputation. (Picture courtesy of Ghazi Rayan MD).

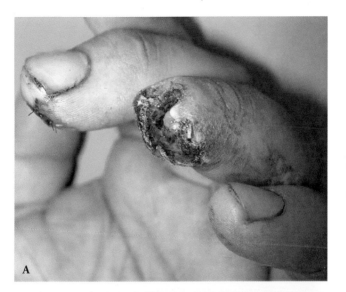

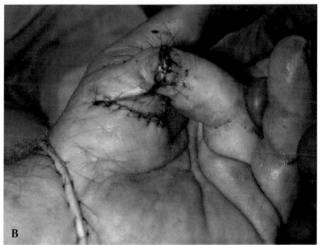

FIGURE 17-3 A–C: Finger tip amputation treated with thenar flap. (*continued*)

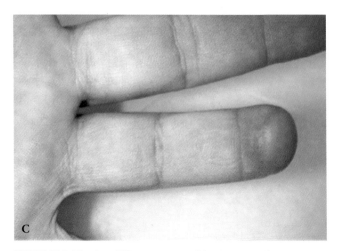

FIGURE 17-3 (*Continued*) (Picture courtesy of Ghazi Rayan MD).

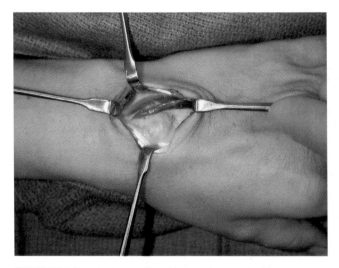

FIGURE 17-4 Dorsal wrist ganglion with anomalous muscle. (Picture courtesy of Ghazi Rayan MD).

utilized for coverage of a thumb tip injury. This procedure entails two longitudinal incisions along the radial and ulnar aspect of the thumb, from injury site to base. As there is independent vascularity of the volar and dorsal skin in the thumb, this large flap can be elevated vulgarly and advanced distally with minimal risk of skin compromise.

Tumors in the subcutaneous tissues of the hand are either benign or malignant. Benign soft tissue tumors are much more common than malignant tumors. The most common tumors and tumor-like conditions encountered in the hand are ganglions (Fig. 17-4), localized villonodular synovitis (soft-tissue giant cell tumors) (Fig. 17-5), lipomas (Fig. 17-6), and inclusion cysts. The most common malignant soft tissue tumor of the subcutaneous space is epithelioid sarcoma. Malignant tumors of the skin, such as squamous cell carcinoma, can invade the subcutaneous space.

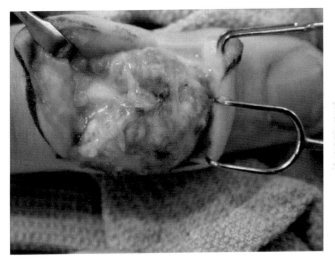

FIGURE 17-5 Localized villonodular synovitis (soft-tissue giant cell tumor of the tendon sheath). (Picture courtesy of Ghazi Rayan MD).

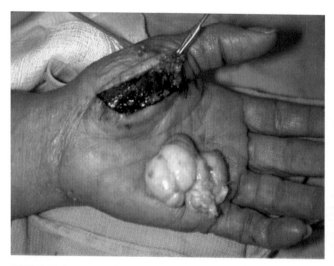

FIGURE 17-6 Lipoma of the thenar aspect of the hand. (Picture courtesy of Ghazi Rayan MD).

Painless benign small masses do not require treatment. Painful or enlarging benign lesions and those that are placing pressure on neurovascular structures can be treated by excision. Malignant tumors should be treated with radical excision or amputation.

CHAPTER 18

Deep Fascia

Physical examination of the palmar fascial complex including digital fascia consists of inspection and palpation. The most common pathological condition of the palmar fascia is Dupuytren disease (DD). This condition is a benign fibro-proliferative disorder in which palpable pathologic nodules and cords develop from the normal fascial structures (Fig.18-1). It is important to differentiate between DD and non-Dupuytren disease. The typical DD is a genetic condition that affects males more than females of northern European descent. It is a bilateral, progressive disorder that leads to digital contracture. DD may be associated with ectopic disease such as dorsal Dupuytren nodules, plantar fibromatosis in the foot, and Peyrones disease in the genitalia. Non-Dupuytren disease is a fibro-proliferation of palmar fascia that follows trauma or surgery. It is nonprogressive, unilateral, and has no genetic, gender, or ethnic predisposition.

CLINICAL CLASSIFICATION OF DUPUYTREN DISEASE

- Early disease (Phase I) produces a *pseudocallus* or thickening of the skin and underlying subcutaneous tissue due to the involvement of the vertical bands of the palmar fascia. This primarily begins around the distal palmar crease, and the skin loses its normal mobility in this area. *Skin pits* may form following contracture of the distal first superficial layer of the split pretendinous band that inserts into the dermis.
- Intermediate disease (Phase II) is characterized by the development of *nodules and cords*, which are pathognomonic of DD (Fig. 18-2). A Dupuytren nodule usually forms as a palpable mass at the distal palmar crease level. It may be transiently painful

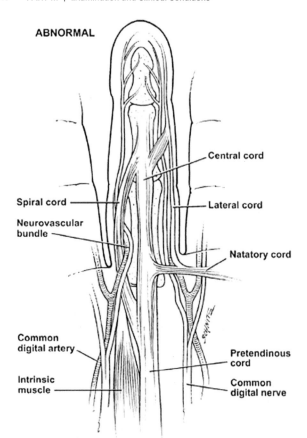

ABNORMAL

Central cord

Spiral cord

Lateral cord

Neurovascular
bundle

Natatory cord

Common
digital artery

Pretendinous
cord

Intrinsic
muscle

Common
digital nerve

FIGURE 18-1 Pathological anatomy of Dupuytren disease in the fingers. (Reproduced from Hughes TB, Mechrefe A, Littler JW, et al. Dupuytren's Disease. *J Amer Soc Surg Hand.* 2003; 3:27–40, Figure 4).

but typically it is painless and may be slightly tender only with direct pressure. The nodule may expand proximally and distally, and thickens forming a cord.

- Advanced disease (Phase III) is characterized by the development of joint and tissue contractures, which are later manifestations of DD (Fig. 18-3).

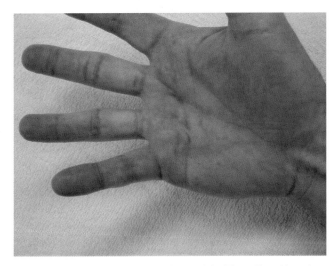

FIGURE 18-2 Early and intermediate phases of the DD manifested by palmar skin thickening in line with the middle finger, palmar skin pit formation, and nodule in line with the small finger and palpable cord formation.

PATHOLOGIC FINDINGS OF DUPUYTREN DISEASE

- The *pretendinous cord* is the most common pathologic tissue in DD. It forms from the normal pretendinous band and most commonly causes a flexion deformity of the metacarpophalangeal (MP) joint (Fig. 18-3).
- The *central cord* is a distal continuation of the pretendinous cord into the digit. In particular it forms from the middle layer of the split pretendinous band. It attaches to the flexor tendon sheath just distal to the proximal interphalangeal (PIP) joint and base of the middle phalanx. It causes MP and PIP joint flexion deformity that may lead in long standing cases to PIP joint contracture.
- The vertical cord is the diseased septum of Legueu and Juvara which departs from the deep surface of the pretendinous cord.
- The *spiral cord* is a palmodigital cord that is made up of four normal structures: the pretendinous band, the spiral band, the lateral digital sheet, and Grayson ligament. As the spiral cord

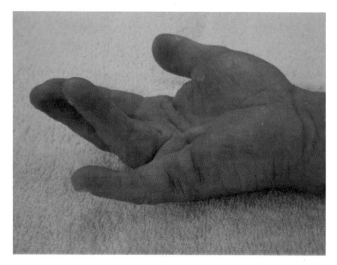

FIGURE 18-3 Pretendinous DD cord in the ring finger.

thickens and contracts, the neurovascular bundle is displaced proximally, centrally, and superficially. This places the neurovascular bundle at a high risk for injury during DD surgery. The spiral cord also causes a PIP joint flexion deformity.

- The *lateral cord* origin is the lateral digital sheet. It is a digital cord but also may be a continuation of the pretendinous cord. It attaches to the skin near Grayson ligament. It causes PIP joint flexion deformity. Rarely, it causes distal interphalangeal (DIP) joint contracture if it extends past the DIP joint.
- The *abductor digiti minimi (ADM) cord* in the small finger is also known as the isolated digital cord. It originates from the musculotendinous area of the ADM near the MP joint and inserts on the ulnar side of the base of the middle phalanx (Fig. 18-4). It causes PIP joint flexion deformity and rarely DIP deformity.
- Proximal and distal commissural cords involve the proximal and distal commissural ligaments and cause thumb–index web space contractures.
- The natatory cord limits the spread of the digits through thickening of the normal natatory ligament at the digital web spaces.

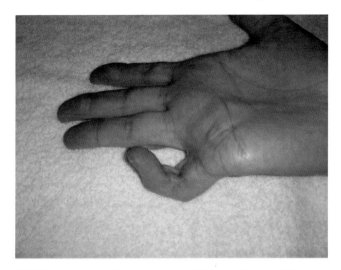

FIGURE 18-4 Isolated digital cord of the small finger arising from ADM muscle insertion.

DIFFERENTIAL DIAGNOSIS

While diagnosing DD in the intermediate and advanced stages (Phases II and III) is easy, this can be difficult in the early stage disease (Phase I) as this may mimic callous formation. Chronic friction in a manual laborer may lead to callous formation and hyperkeratosis near the distal palmar crease that simulates early DD. Pulley rupture or attenuation with the flexor tendon bowstringing as in climbers may mimic a Dupuytren cord. Dupuytren nodules, in contrast, must be distinguished from other subcutaneous masses including ganglion cyst, epidermoid inclusion cyst in the palm, and giant cell tumor of tendon sheath. Lastly DD must be differentiated from malignant soft tissue tumors such as epithelioid sarcoma.

CLINICAL PRESENTATION

- In the early Phase I of the disease the diagnosis of the condition can be difficult but patients do not have any symptoms.

- In the intermediate Phase II of the disease the diagnosis of the condition is much easier. The patient also is usually asymptomatic unless the nodule or vertical cord contributes to the development of painful stenosing tenosynovitis and rarely triggering of the fingers.
- In the advanced Phase III of the disease the digital flexion deformity becomes more than a nuisance when it is more than 30 degrees at the MP and 15 degrees at the PIP joint.
- Positive tabletop test: the palm and fingers cannot be placed flat on a table simultaneously due to joint and tissue contractures.
- Joint contractures are most common at the MP followed by the PIP and least common at the DIP joint. Typically when these contractures cause functional deficits such as inability to put one's hand in a pocket or difficulty with fine motor skills, the patient seeks treatment.

TREATMENT OPTIONS

- Nonsurgical treatment options: Observation is indicated if the deformity does not interfere with patient's function. The two nonsurgical techniques for DD are minimally invasive and can be office based and aimed at partially correcting the deformity without removing the diseased tissue. The indication for this intervention is typically a patient with dysfunction from a disease limited to the palm with MP joint deformity.

   The first, most established method is percutaneous needle fasciotomy. This technique utilizes local anesthesia and needle punctures of the longitudinal cord, through multiple portals, followed by manipulation to rupture the cord. This treatment usually improves the deformity. Early results are promising with this technique although the rapidity of disease recurrence is a concern.

   The second method is enzymatic injection into the cord which is intended to weaken the cord. This is followed by the application of mechanical force 24 hours later to extend the finger, thus rupturing the cord. Early results are promising, but some question remains about recurrence and cost.

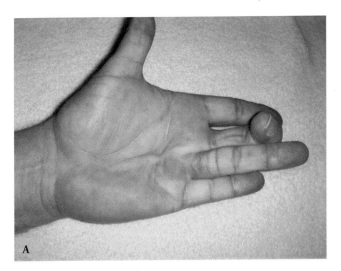

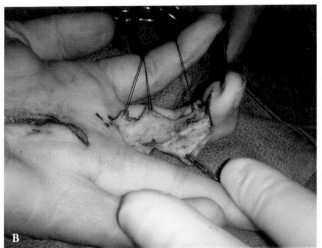

FIGURE 18-5 A–C: Pre and intraoperative pictures of DD tissue. Preoperative pretendinous cord of the ring and digital cord of the middle (**A**), intraoperative appearance (**B**). (*continued*)

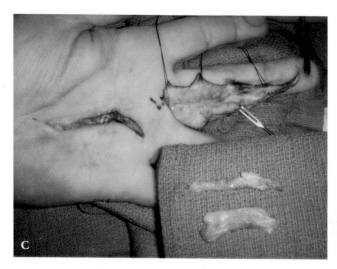

FIGURE 18-5 (*Continued*) and intraoperative appearance after partial fasciectomy (**C**). (All pictures provided by Ghazi Rayan MD).

- Surgical treatment has the objective of removing the diseased tissue, which is the traditional method of treating advanced and recurrent DD (Fig. 18-5). Surgical indications include an MP joint contracture of 30 degrees or more and/or PIP joint contracture of more than 10 degrees. Open limited fasciectomy by selectively removing the diseased tissue remains the most widely used treatment for DD (Fig. 18-5A–C). This involves operative excision of the diseased tissue, preserving any uninvolved fascial and neurovascular tissue.

CHAPTER 19

Hand Spaces

There are numerous bony and soft tissue structures that are confined within the hand and digits. During each hand examination, isolating and identifying each structure and assessing its function is important for making an accurate diagnosis. Knowing the locations and contents of the various hand spaces is critical when evaluating and treating many conditions affecting the hand and forearm. The basic examination for hand space disorders mandates appraisal of both intrinsic and extrinsic tendon function, muscle function, joint stability and range of motion, and the neurological and vascular status of the hand. Hand spaces can be involved in traumatic, infectious, inflammatory, and neoplastic conditions.

TRAUMA

Hand spaces can be disrupted by traumatic events such as penetrating and crushing injuries, blunt trauma, fractures, and dislocations. Injuries of hand spaces do not require special treatment other than treating the primary condition and adequate wound irrigation to prevent infection. In certain cases of flexor tendon lacerations in zone 2 where both the flexor digitorum superficialis and flexor digitorum profundus are contained within the same tendon sheath, repairing the synovial sheath is done if feasible.

ACUTE INFECTIONS

Probably the most germane clinical application for knowing the anatomy of hand spaces is in the area of treating hand infections. Hand infections may affect any or many of the various hand spaces and can be caused by various pathogens, most usually bacterial and most often *Staphylococcus aureus*. If their diagnosis and treatment are delayed the results may be catastrophic to future hand function and occasionally result in amputation and even septicemia that jeopardizes the patient's life.

Flexor Tendon Sheath Infection

This is known as septic or pyogenic flexor tenosynovitis. The flexor tendon sheath of the digits is a closed space that acquires infection either from penetrating injury or hematogenous spread. When a bacterial contamination occurs in this sterile environment, usually from an open injury, infection sets in and the symptoms and signs of septic tenosynovitis become visible acutely and progresses rapidly. Kanavel described the four cardinal signs associated with this condition: (i) flexed posture of the finger, (ii) symmetric swelling of the digit, (iii) excessive tenderness along the course of the flexor tendon sheath, and (iv) excruciating pain on passively extending the involved digit, especially at the proximal aspect of the sheath (Fig. 19-1).

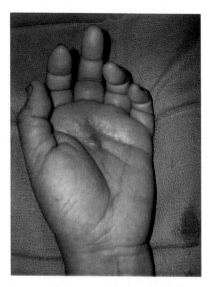

FIGURE 19-1 Purulent flexor tenosynovitis of the middle finger. There is diffuse swelling in the palm and abnormal posture of the finger. (Picture is courtesy of Ghazi Rayan MD).

Accurate diagnosis and early treatment is imperative for achieving satisfactory outcome and hand function. When this infection is identified early, within 24 hours of onset, admission to the hospital, splinting, elevation, and appropriate IV antibiotics may halt the spread of infection. If the patient does not respond to nonoperative treatment measures or the infection is severe or delayed, then surgical drainage of the tendon sheath is critical for controlling the infection. The presence of purulence within the tendon sheath will interfere with tendon vascularity and nutrition provided by vincular vessels and synovial fluid. Failure to drain the sheath will result in tendon necrosis and subsequent exuberant amount of scarring with peritendinous adhesions to the surrounding tissue and limitation of digital motion and hand function. Knowing the anatomical extent of the tendon sheath helps in surgical planning of skin incisions.

Bursal Infection

Patients with infection of the radial or ulnar bursa present with pain, swelling, erythema, and possible fever. There is tenderness along the infected bursa and in the corresponding finger if digital extension occurs. Sometimes the infection may spread between the two bursae through a communication or affect Parona space superficial to the pronator quadratus muscle taking the appearance of a "horseshoe" abscess at the wrist or distal forearm. Surgical debridement should be instituted urgently. The treating surgeon must have intimate knowledge of the anatomical structures within these compartments and the important neurovascular structures in proximity, which require protection.

Deep Space Infections

Deep space infections occur either from open trauma or hematogenous spread. Occasionally, infections that develop on the volar aspect of the hand extend dorsally through the digital web space forming a collar-button abscess. When similar infection involves the first web space it may form a thenar space abscess. Web space infections of the hand typically are associated with swelling both volarly and dorsally and the fingers are abducted (Fig. 19-2). Any attempt at digital motion elicits severe pain. Deep palmar space infections can develop as an extension from septic tenosynovitis and visa versa. This infection

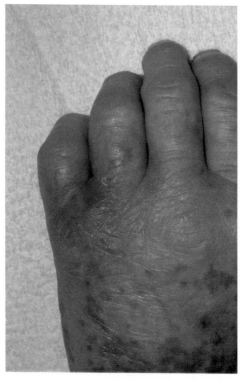

FIGURE 19-2 Deep web space infection with diffuse swelling and erythema of the fourth web space. (Picture is courtesy of Ghazi Rayan MD).

is associated with severe pain and swelling in the mid-palm that obliterates the normal concavity of the hand. Infections of all deep spaces require IV antibiotics and drainage. Web space infections should be drained through both volar and dorsal incisions, with care to protect the nearby important anatomical structures.

Superficial Space Infections

These may affect the subcutaneous space of the dorsum of the hand (Fig. 19-3A) or the palmar subcutaneous space (Fig. 19-3B).

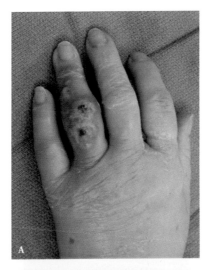

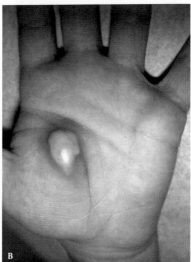

FIGURE 19-3 Dorsal subcutaneous space infection (**A**) and palmar subcutaneous space infection (**B**) with abscess formation. (Pictures are courtesy of Ghazi Rayan MD).

Pulp Space Infection (Felon)

A felon is a bacterial infection of the fingertip pulp, usually caused by penetrating trauma, which causes an abscess trapped by the fibrous bands connecting the periosteum and the dermis (Fig. 19-4). Because these small compartments do not expand, the finger pulp becomes swollen with severe throbbing pain that interferes with patients sleep and may be refractory to rest, elevation, and even pain medication. As in most hand infections the most common offending organism is *Staph aureus*, and the treatment includes appropriate antibiotics and drainage by dividing all bands and decompressing the affected compartments. This condition should not be confused with herpetic whitlow, which is a viral infection of the finger pulp that is not treated surgically.

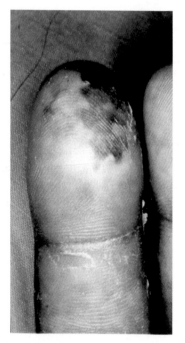

FIGURE 19-4 Felon of the pulp space with late diagnosis and early skin necrosis. (Picture is courtesy of Ghazi Rayan MD).

INFLAMMATORY CONDITIONS

Various inflammatory conditions such as rheumatoid arthritis, systemic lupus erythematosus (Fig. 19-5A and B), psoriasis, and colitis may cause diffuse proliferative flexor or extensor tenosynovitis affecting the digits, hand, and distal forearm. In severe inflammatory tenosynovitis

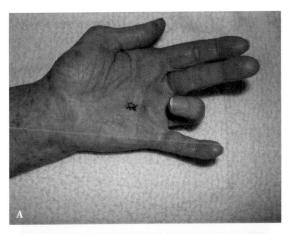

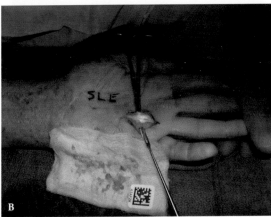

FIGURE 19-5 Inflammatory tenosynovitis in a patient with systemic lupus presented with swelling and triggering (**A**) that was treated with tenosynovectomy (**B**). (Pictures are courtesy of Ghazi Rayan MD).

the entire palmar sheath or bursal sac becomes diffusely enlarged with resultant pain and limitation of active but not passive flexion. Similar findings are encountered on the dorsum of the wrist. Sometimes, the swelling in the volar wrist and forearm may compress adjacent structures such as the median nerve causing carpal tunnel syndrome. Chronic untreated tenosynovitis, especially dorsally, may infiltrate extensor tendons and result in tendon rupture (Fig. 19-6A and B). Nonoperative treatment of the primary disease often controls the

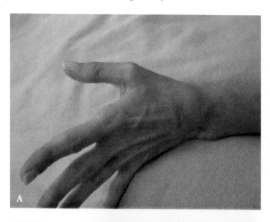

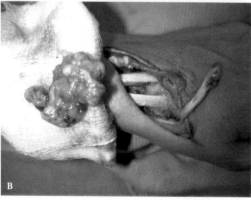

FIGURE 19-6 Inflammatory tenosynovitis of the dorsum of the wrist with extensor pollicis longus (EPL) tendon rupture (**A**) that was treated with tenosynovectomy and tendon transfers (**B**). (Pictures are courtesy of Ghazi Rayan MD).

tenosynovitis. Chronic recalcitrant conditions should be treated by tenosynovectomy to decrease swelling, control pain, restore motion, and prevent rupture. Invasive tendon rupture requires surgical reconstruction. Gouty tenosynovitis is due to calcium urate crystal deposition in soft tissues including tenosynovium (Fig. 19-7A and B).

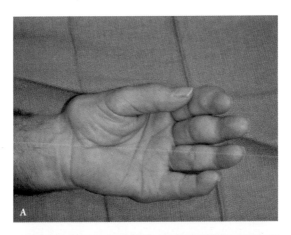

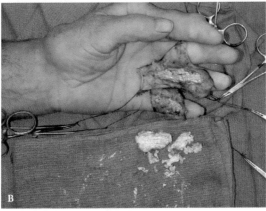

FIGURE 19-7 Patient with gouty flexor tenosynovitis and gouty arthritis (**A**) that was treated by debridement of the gouty tophaceous deposits (**B**) from the involved tenosynovium. (Pictures are courtesy of Ghazi Rayan MD).

Carpal tunnel syndrome can be caused by flexor tenosynovitis. The treatment is decompression of the median nerve and flexor tenosynovectomy.

TUMORS

Most tumors of the hand are benign. These tumors usually enlarge within a compartment of the hand and encroach upon hand spaces. The most common soft tissue tumor affecting the tenosynovium is villonodular synovitis, which may be either diffuse or localized which is also known as giant cell tumor of tendon sheath. Malignant bony and soft tissue tumors of the hand are exceedingly rare. When present these often infiltrate adjacent compartments including hand spaces and tendon sheaths. Asymptomatic benign tumors may be observed; however, when symptomatic they can be excised, with preservation of vital structures. Malignant tumors are treated with radical excision including the entire compartment or amputation.

CHAPTER 20

Vascular System

Vascular system disorders can be classified into acute or chronic. Chronic vascular conditions include thrombotic disorders, aneurysms, or vasospastic disorders. Understanding the anatomy and conducting a thorough physical examination allows an accurate diagnosis to be made, which in turn ensures that appropriate treatment will be offered. Vascular diseases share the common manifestations of pain and ischemia in the hand or digit. A history of smoking, using vibratory tools, connective tissue disorders, atherosclerosis, and cardiac disease should be obtained.

VASCULAR ASSESSMENT

A history of penetrating trauma and pulsatile bleeding is the most common presentation with arterial laceration. Arterial injury may occur from acute blunt trauma or repetitive trauma over a period of time. The onset of pain and color changes in the hand and factors which provoke and relieve them should be noted. There may or may not be ischemia to the involved hand or digit due to the dual blood supply to the hand and fingers, especially if only one artery is injured. However, if there is an anomalous incomplete palmar arterial arch or prior injury to one artery ischemia to the hand may ensue. Injury to both digital arteries will render a finger ischemic.

When a patient is initially examined, often the arterial injury may not be associated with bleeding, either due to vessel lumen contraction, clot formation, or by prior emergency wound management. The wound should only be explored with proximal vessel control using the proper instruments and adequate anesthesia, lighting, and magnification. Typically this is best done in an operating room setting and not in the emergency room. There is little information to be obtained from attempting to explore a wound in the emergency room.

If the patient had previous placement of a temporary tourniquet or pressure dressing with a history of pulsatile bleeding, using a blood pressure cuff allows removal of all dressings and thorough evaluation of the injury. The blood pressure cuff can be placed on the proximal arm and kept inflated while the field dressing or tourniquet is removed in the operating room. Wound examination and irrigation can then be performed. If pulsatile bleeding is encountered, the cuff can be inflated to 50–100 mm Hg above systolic pressure to stop arterial inflow. Other clues during examination that may confirm the presence of an arterial injury, for example to the ulnar artery at the wrist, are laceration to the flexor carpi ulnaris tendon and ulnar nerve. These are suggested by wrist flexion weakness and loss of sensory function in the ring and small fingers, respectively. Both of these structures are ulnar to the ulnar artery at the wrist level. Injury to the radial artery on the other hand may be associated with flexor carpi radialis tendon laceration which is located ulnar to the radial artery. Another clue for possible arterial injury is laceration to the abductor pollicis longus, which is radial to the artery at the wrist. Radial artery injury may also be suggested by loss of sensory function of the palmar cutaneous branch of the median nerve (over the thenar area) which is located just ulnar to the flexor carpi radialis tendon. This may be associated with damage to a branch of the superficial radial nerve which gives sensation along the radial thumb base.

In the digits, ischemia can occur when both digital arteries are severed. This is often associated with laceration of digital flexor tendons. In the digit, the nerves are superficial to the arteries. Hence loss of sensation to one or both sides of the digit is usually associated with arterial injury. Occasionally, a digit may survive for a short time on flow from dorsal digital arterial branches. The thumb may survive if both digital arteries are severed from the circulation of the dorsal digital artery. However, this circulation may not be optimal and the digital arteries should be repaired.

Palpation for pulses although helpful is not the most reliable method for diagnosing arterial injuries. Capillary refill in the affected digit does not exclude arterial injury as this may be present due to collateral vessels. Allen test is very useful to assess arterial injury. Failure to achieve flow to the hand after release of the radial artery indicates loss of continuity of the radial or ulnar artery. This test can be done on the fingers with pressure applied and released over the radial and ulnar digital arteries in a similar manner.

Vascular injury may occur due to closed blunt trauma such as a crush injury with bleeding from within a fracture. When the external pressure around the small vessels and capillaries compromises blood flow, muscle and nerve ischemia can occur. Bleeding into a muscle compartment from a fracture can lead to increased compartment pressures and acute compartment syndrome. Manifestations of compartment syndrome include pain out of proportion to the apparent injury, a tense muscle compartment, pain with passive stretch of the digits or muscle in question, and limited active motion. Diminished pulse and possible pallor of the extremity are less reliable findings.

In the absence of acute trauma, ischemia may occur either from emboli that dislodge from an intra-arterial thrombus and lodge in the digital arteries. This may be associated with vasospasm from sympathetic overactivity. Allen test may reveal occlusion of the radial (prior cannulation) or ulnar (blunt trauma) artery. Cardiac examination may reveal a more central cause of thromboembolism such as a mural thrombus. Mural thrombi may be from atrial fibrillation, myocardial infarction, heart valve abnormalities and infections, or prosthetic valves. These cause over two-third of all upper extremity emboli.

Patients affected with vasospastic disorders such as Raynaud disease often exhibit a characteristic color change pattern in the digits. The finger becomes white (pallor) due to ischemia which is often initiated by cold exposure or emotional distress. Next the fingers take on a bluish tint due to venous congestion (cyanosis) and as the fingers recover blood flow they become red from vasodilatation (hyperemia). This is usually associated with intense burning pain. If left untreated, Raynaud disease can cause ischemic necrosis of the finger tips.

Upper extremity deep venous thrombosis (DVT) is being recognized with increasing frequency. This diagnosis often presents with upper extremity pain, hand swelling, cyanosis, edema, and muscle weakness. Diagnosis can be made by appropriate clinical examination.

Various radiologic studies can determine whether venous thrombosis or an arterial injury and occlusion have occurred. These may be performed as venography or the most commonly used arteriogram. An arteriogram is done by injecting contrast material or dye proximal to the injury site, such as the brachial artery for hand injuries, followed by sequential X-rays. Other studies that can be used are MRI/angiography and ultrasound. Compartment pressures can be measured with various commercially available devices or by simply assembling a system in the emergency department (Fig. 20-1). Typically a pressure above 30 mm Hg in a normotensive patient is considered synonymous with a diagnosis of compartment syndrome.

Digital pulse volume recording (PVR), termed digital plethysmography, is used in vasospastic disorders before and after cold stress or ice immersion of the fingers. If a sympathetic block to the digits greatly improves PVR after cold immersion, this is diagnostic of vasospastic disease. Ultrasound techniques for arterial and venous disease are now being employed in some centers but diagnostic accuracy is dependent on technique and ultrasonographer experience. Doppler studies can be readily performed at bedside to

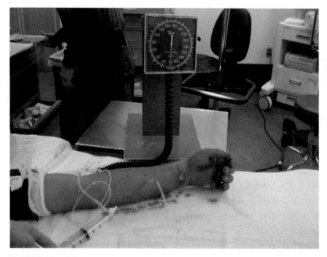

FIGURE 20-1 Whiteside method of measuring the compartment pressure. (Picture courtesy of Ghazi Rayan MD).

detect arterial flow but they are prone to error especially in atherosclerotic vessels. Skin temperature measurements are another way to assess adequate arterial flow and have been primarily used in free flap monitoring and replantation.

ACUTE ARTERIAL LACERATION

Complete arterial lacerations may not continuously bleed as the muscular intimal layer contracts and vasospasm, followed by thrombosis, may stop bleeding. Partial arterial lacerations, on the other hand, will produce continued pulsatile bleeding as the arterial ends cannot contract, leaving the arterial laceration open. Arterial repair is mandatory if there is ischemia of the affected part. Uncontrolled bleeding represents a surgical emergency. Ischemia lasting more than 4–6 hours in an extremity with muscles affected will predispose to compartment syndrome. Vessels are repaired in the course of repairing-associated nerve or tendon injuries. Isolated digital artery, radial, or ulnar artery repairs remain controversial especially if ischemia is not present. Microvascular repair in experienced hands has been shown to approach patency rates greater than 90%.

ACUTE COMPARTMENT SYNDROME

Compartment syndromes in the hand and forearm are due to ischemia followed by edema, which becomes a vicious cycle that occurs when there is a rapid rise in the hand or forearm compartment pressure. Bleeding into a muscle compartment from fractures can lead to increased compartment pressures. Constrictive casts and tight splints or dressings may predispose a patient to acute compartment syndrome. A compartment syndrome is a surgical emergency, which requires immediate fasciotomy.

ARTERIAL THROMBOSIS/ THROMBOEMBOLIC DISEASE

The most common thrombotic disorder in the hand is that of the ulnar artery, called hypothenar hammer syndrome. The patient complaints of pain in the ulnar aspect of the hand often associated with numbness in the ulnar nerve distribution. Thrombosis of the artery occurs in Guyon canal and arterial swelling may cause compression of the ulnar nerve. Ischemia occurs either from emboli that break off from the intra-arterial clot and lodge in the digital arteries or due to vasospasm from sympathetic overtone. While any digit can have emboli from ulnar artery thrombosis, the ring finger is most typically affected. Examination reveals tenderness to palpation at Guyon canal along with lack of flow from the ulnar artery on Allen test. An angiogram will confirm the diagnosis. Treatment is directed to predisposing factors such as cessation of smoking and avoiding repeated trauma to the ulnar aspect of the hand along with the use of vasodilators. Surgical reconstruction may be appropriate if non-operative interventions fail to resolve symptoms. Radial artery thrombosis may be iatrogenic following placement of an arterial line or due to atherosclerosis (Fig. 20-2 A and B).

Burgers disease is another vascular occlusive disease named thromboangiitis obliterans. It affects more males who are heavy smokers. Ischemic ulcers followed by necrosis and fingertip amputations are common (Fig. 20-3).

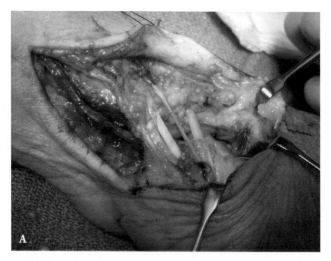

FIGURE 20-2 Atherosclerotic thrombosis of the radial artery in the wrist and hand before (**A**) and after resection and interposition vein grafting (**B**). (*continued*)

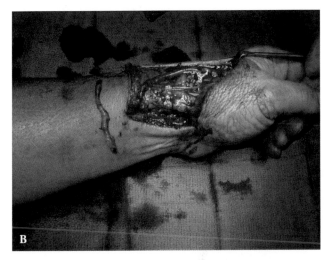

FIGURE 20-2 (*Continued*) (Pictures courtesy of Ghazi Rayan MD).

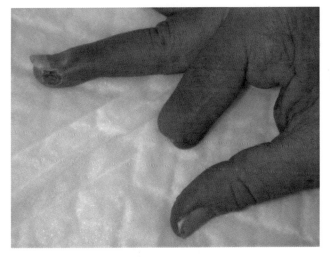

FIGURE 20-3 Ischemic ulcer of the middle and post amputation of the index finger in a patient with Burger disease. (Picture courtesy of Ghazi Rayan MD).

A common origin of digital emboli is a thrombus from the radial artery that has formed after cannulation for arterial lines. If the thrombus formation is recognized early, often by Allen testing, non-operative management can be administered, such as anticoagulation with occasional local thrombolytic therapy. If these measures are ineffective and ischemia or digital emboli ensue, then thrombectomy or more appropriately resection of the damaged arterial segment may be indicated. If the segment is large an interposition graft may be needed.

Emboli may lodge in the hand from distant sites with the subclavian artery and the heart considered the most common source (Fig. 20-4A–B). Patients will complain of acute pain and digital pallor if there is ischemia and no collateral flow. If recognized early, these conditions can be treated with anti-thrombolytic agents and

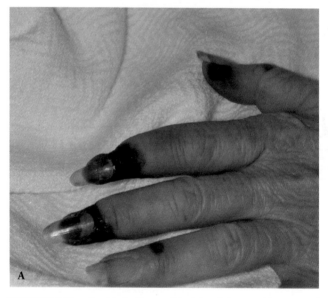

FIGURE 20-4 Thromboembolic disease of the left radial artery and gangrene of the radial fingers (**A**) and similar disease of both radial and ulnar arteries of the right hand (**B**). (*continued*)

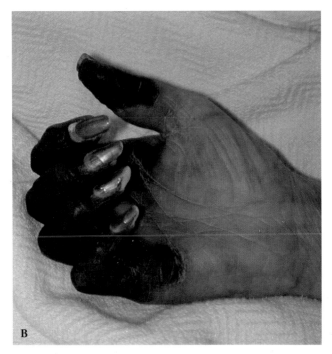

B

FIGURE 20-4 (*Continued*) (Pictures courtesy of Ghazi Rayan MD).

anti-coagulation along with a full cardiac work-up to find the origin of the thrombus. If non-operative management is ineffective, thrombectomy or resection of the diseased segment should be performed along with interposition vein grafting.

ANEURYSMS

Aneurysms may develop in arteries of the forearm and wrist. Most commonly, the ulnar artery is affected. The aneurysm can be either a true or false aneurysm (Fig. 20-5A–C). True aneurysms involve all three layers of the artery – intima, media, and adventitia. They are usually the result of blunt injury and are likely to produce emboli. False aneurysms result from penetrating trauma such as knife

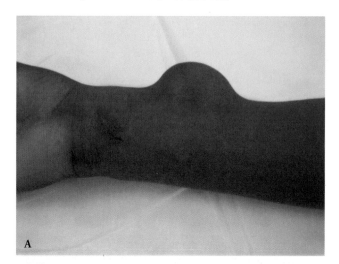

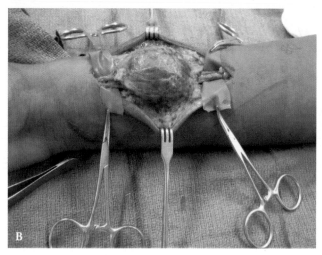

FIGURE 20-5 False aneurysm of the radial artery following penetrating injury of the forearm (**A**). Intraoperative appearance of the aneurysm before (**B**) and (**C**) following resection and interposition vein grafting. (*continued*)

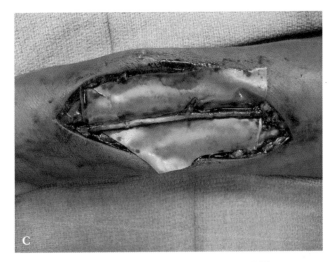

FIGURE 20-5 (*Continued*) (Pictures courtesy of Ghazi Rayan MD).

wounds or cannulation injuries. A false aneurysm forms when there is bleeding outside of the wall of the artery. A hematoma then forms an outside endothelial wall. The lining of the false aneurysm does not contain a media or intimal layer. Both types of aneurysms typically present as a painful pulsatile mass. Surgery is the only recommended treatment to decrease pain, improve blood flow, prevent emboli to distal sites, and most importantly rupture the aneurysm.

RAYNAUD DISEASE

The most common name associated with vasospastic disorders of the hand is that of Raynaud. This is a primary vasospastic disorder of unknown etiology called Raynaud disease (Fig. 20-6). The most common demographic group affected is young women who typically have bilateral disease. Raynaud phenomenon is the term used when the patient has identifiable cause for the vasospastic symptoms. Examples include collagen vascular disease

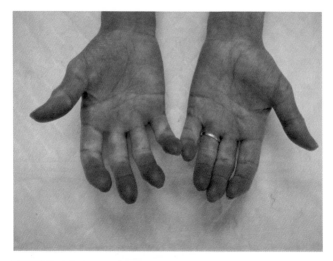

FIGURE 20-6 Typical discoloration of both hands digits in patient with Raynaud disease. (Picture courtesy of Ghazi Rayan MD).

such as scleroderma and rheumatoid arthritis, frostbite, neurologic disorders, and smoking. Any gender and age group can be affected and the findings may be limited to one hand. Diagnosis is made by history, physical examination, and ancillary tests. Angiogram is rarely indicated because it is often normal. In advanced cases an angiogram may show tapering off of the digital vessels as the flow decreases to the finger tips. Cold stress testing is helpful in the diagnosis.

Initial treatment is preventive directed toward protection of the hands from cold exposure and eliminating factors that would increase digital spasm such as using caffeine and nicotine. Oral vasodilating agents such as calcium channel blockers, aspirin (block platelet aggregation), and sidenifil (Viagra) have also been used. Topical agents such as nitropaste have been tried with mixed results. If these agents are ineffective and the patient shows improvement of PVR with sympathetic block, then microscopic digital sympathectomy has been effective in a significant segment of this patient population.

VENOUS OCCLUSION

Upper extremity DVT may be the result of trauma, systemic disease, or hypercoagulable states. Symptoms and signs depend on the existing collateral vessels and the appropriateness of mechanisms that control vasomotor/autonomic function. Due to the vast number of distal venous channels, DVT in the hand usually does not pose a clinical problem. However, if the cephalic or basilic vein, which starts at the wrist, becomes thrombosed, symptoms can result. Diagnosis is made by appropriate clinical examination and most often by venography. Treatment is usually supportive and seldom surgical.

CHAPTER 21

Peripheral Nervous System

GENERAL NERVE EXAMINATION

Peripheral nerve examination is an essential component of a thorough hand and upper extremity evaluation. This is conducted in the settings of both acute injury and elective conditions. During preliminary evaluation of any acute injury it is critical to assess the status of the upper extremity peripheral nerves. A complete nerve examination should be performed in the trauma bay before and after any fracture reduction. Few things are more disconcerting than performing a fracture manipulation and then learning that there is a nerve deficit without knowledge of the nerve function prior to fracture treatment.

Performing a sensory examination of the hand relies on the understanding of its innervation patterns. While there is some dermatomal overlap among different sensory nerves, there are certain predominant areas of innervation that can reliably test the integrity of each peripheral nerve in the hand. The predominant sensory zone for the radial nerve is in the dorsal first web space, the median nerve at the volar tip of the index finger, and the ulnar nerve at the volar tip of the small finger (Fig. 21-1).

Initial sensory evaluation may begin with the assessment of light touch perception. However, this is an imprecise method of evaluating nerve integrity. A more exact appraisal of nerve injury is the two-point discrimination test, which measures innervation density. A blunt-tipped caliper (Fig. 21-2) is used to assess the minimum distance between the two points of the caliper that a patient can distinguish. An alternative to a caliper would be a paper clip (Fig. 21-3). A two-point discrimination test of 5 mm at the fingertip is considered normal and confirms an intact sensory nerve function. A two-point discrimination test greater than 12 mm indicates nerve laceration or damage

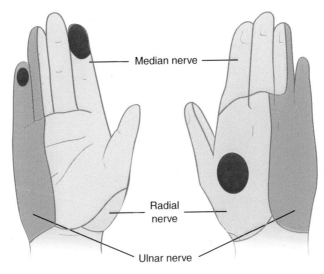

FIGURE 21-1 Sensory zones of peripheral nerves in the hand.

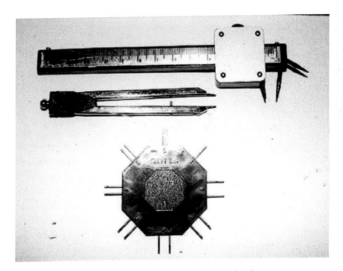

FIGURE 21-2 Calipers for measuring two-point discrimination.

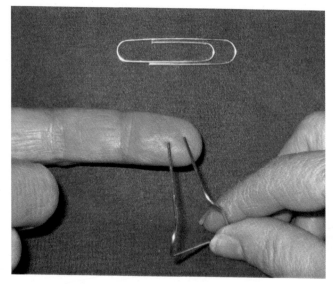

FIGURE 21-3 A paper clip is a handy tool for measuring two-point discrimination.

from severe compression. A Semmes–Weinstein monofilament test is a threshold test that is done by a hand therapist. Progressively larger monofilaments are applied to the digit to assess the size of the filament necessary for the patient to appreciate the pressure. Threshold tests are more sensitive for compressive neuropathy.

Active thumb interphalangeal (IP) joint extension is a reliable test for assessing radial nerve motor function, including the posterior interosseous nerve (PIN). Median nerve motor function can be tested by assessing thumb abduction or opposition, which is a function of its recurrent motor branch. Additionally median nerve function is assessed by the ability to make an "O" or the OK sign by flexion of thumb IP and index distal interphalangeal joints, which is the function of the anterior interosseous nerve (AIN). Index finger abduction is the function of the first dorsal interosseous muscle, which is innervated by the ulnar nerve. In a few seconds all three nerves can be evaluated (Fig. 21-4A–C) by asking the patient to make a thumb up

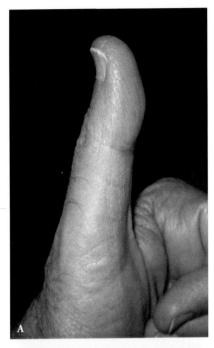

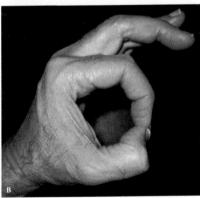

FIGURE 21-4 Thumb extension (radial nerve, i.e., AIN) (**A**), OK or O sign (median nerve, i.e., AIN) (**B**), and resistive pinching (ulnar nerve) (**C**). (*continued*)

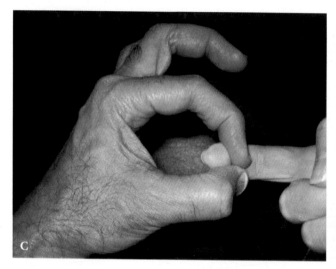

FIGURE 21-4 (Continued)

sign (extensor pollicis longus = radial), an O or OK sign [flexor pollicis longus, flexor digitorum profundus = median anterior interosseus nerve (AIN)], and resist breaking up the O sign (first dorsal interosseous and adductor pollicis muscles P = ulnar nerve).

PEDIATRIC NERVE CONDITIONS

The most common peripheral nerve problem in newborns is an injury to the brachial plexus during delivery. The condition is termed "birth palsy" or Erb palsy and occurs in 0.1%–0.5% of live births. Risk factors for brachial plexus injury include increased birth weight (as seen with gestational diabetes), shoulder dystocia, prolonged labor, and fetal distress during labor. Examination of the newborn with a brachial plexus injury is focused on determining the severity (pre- or post-ganglionic injury), level of the injury (roots, trunks, cords) and extent (number of cervical roots) affected (Fig. 21-5). In Erb palsy, which is an upper-trunk lesion (C5–C6, +/−C7), the child presents

Brachial plexus palsy injuries

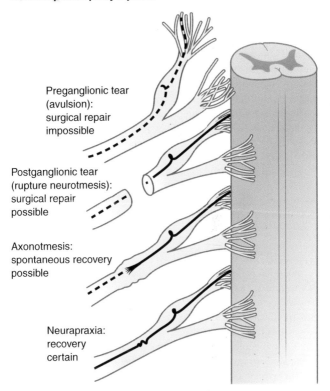

Preganglionic tear
(avulsion):
surgical repair
impossible

Postganglionic tear
(rupture neurotmesis):
surgical repair
possible

Axonotmesis:
spontaneous recovery
possible

Neurapraxia:
recovery
certain

FIGURE 21-5 A severe traction injury to the brachial plexus may cause nerve injuries of varying severity in the same plexus. These include avulsion of the nerve root from the spinal cord (nonrepairable), extraforaminal rupture of the root or trunk (surgically repairable), and intraneural rupture of fascicles (some spontaneous recovery possible).

with an internally rotated, adducted limb with the forearm in pronation and the wrist in flexion (the "waiter's tip" position). This is the most common pattern of birth plexus injury. The second most common is a complete palsy (C5-T1), and these children present with a flail limb. Lower-trunk injuries (C8-T1) are uncommon and patients have severe hand paralysis with spared elbow and shoulder function.

Injuries proximal to the dorsal root ganglion (pre-ganglionic) are associated with injury to the cervical sympathetic ganglion. This plexus injury is accompanied by Horner syndrome (pupillary constriction or miosis), lowering of the eyelid to the level of the pupil (ptosis), sinking of the eyeball within the socket (enophthalmos), and dry face (anhidrosis) due to the absence of sweating. Pre-ganglionic injuries have a poorer prognosis than those distal to the dorsal root ganglion. The treatment of brachial plexus injuries includes early observation and joint contracture prevention. If recovery does not begin by 3 to 4 months, surgical exploration of the plexus may be necessary. In patients with chronic plexopathy, late reconstruction by tendon transfers to restore shoulder abduction and elbow flexion will be indicated.

TRAUMATIC NERVE INJURIES

Traumatic nerve injuries are most often caused by lacerations that lead to motor and/or sensory deficit. Other nerve injuries may be caused by traction or compression. Nerve injuries can be classified into three categories. *Neurapraxia* is the transient disruption of axonal transport and conductivity within the nerve. The nerve fibers remain intact and recovery is usually rapid and complete. *Axonotmesis* occurs when there is disruption of the nerve fibers, but the axonal sheath remains intact. Distal to the site of the injury, the nerve undergoes Wallerian degeneration. Recovery is inconsistent and much slower, occurring at a rate of approximately 1 mm/day. *Neurotmesis* involves complete disruption of the nerve fibers and the sheath. No recovery is expected without surgical repair.

Nerve lacerations require exploration and repair. Blast injuries, such as from gunshot wounds, should be initially observed. When these are explored, all damaged tissue at the zone of injury must be resected prior to nerve repair. Neurorrhaphy involves the suturing of the epineurium of the two lacerated nerve ends without tension at the repair site. In certain circumstances this will require the use of an interposition nerve graft.

Adult brachial plexus lesions occur either from penetrating injury (such as a knife) or from traction (such as in a motorcycle accident). Evaluation is similar to that in the infants with birth palsy. Treatment options include nerve exploration and repair (for lacerations), nerve grafting (for post-ganglionic traction injuries that do not spontaneously recover), nerve transfers, and in chronic cases muscle transfers.

TUMORS

Neoplasms within nerves are most often benign in nature. The most common benign nerve tumor of the upper extremity is neurolemmoma (also known as a schwannoma). This benign tumor arises from the Schwann cells and myelin tissue, can be easily removed, and may be associated with a positive Tinels sign, that is, percussion along the nerve with the examiner's index and middle fingers. Elicitation of paresthesias in the distribution of the specific nerve constitutes a positive test and an indication of nerve dysfunction.

Neurofibromas arise from the nerve fascicles. They are benign tumors that may be associated with neurofibromatosis although solitary neurofibromas can be encountered in the hand. Excision when necessary will result in a nerve deficit that requires reconstruction. Lipofibromatous hamartomas are benign lesions that arise from the fibrous and adipose tissue within the epineurium. When affecting the median nerve in the carpal tunnel the treatment is decompression. Excision of these lesions leads to significant deficits and is performed under rare circumstances.

NERVE COMPRESSION

A common source of nerve dysfunction in the hand is compressive neuropathy. The most common of these disorders is carpal tunnel syndrome (CTS). Patients with CTS complain of paresthesias and sometime pain in the hand. Symptoms are frequently nocturnal. In severe cases the patient has thenar muscle atrophy and absent or markedly increased two-point discrimination. Provocative tests that can help making the diagnosis are Tinel test, Phalen test, and Durkan carpal compression test (Chapter 14). Carpal tunnel

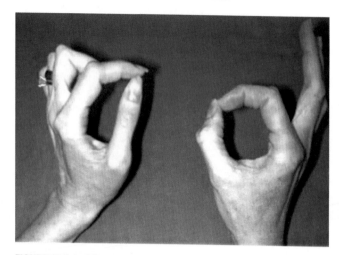

FIGURE 21-6 Inability to make OK sign in AIN palsy. (Picture courtesy of Ghazi Rayan MD).

syndrome can be treated with night splinting, corticosteroid injection into the carpal tunnel, or by surgical release of the transverse carpal ligament. Rarely, the median nerve can be compressed proximal to the elbow by the ligament of Struthers that attaches to the supracondylar process of the humerus or distal to the elbow as it passes through the two heads of the pronator teres muscle (pronator syndrome). In AIN syndrome there is paralysis of the flexor digitorum profundus and flexor pollicis longus tendons of the index and thumb, respectively, with loss of the patient's ability to make the OK sign (Fig. 21-6).

Cubital tunnel syndrome is the second most common compressive neuropathy in the upper extremity. It involves compression of the ulnar nerve at the elbow. The patient complains of paresthesias and hypoesthesia and later anesthesia in the ulnar aspect of the ring finger and small fingers, along with hand weakness due to intrinsic muscle atrophy in advanced stages. There is a positive Tinel sign over the ulnar nerve in the cubital tunnel and a positive, elbow flexion test (Chapter 14). In severe ulnar nerve palsy the patient has the following signs: 1) Froment sign (flexing the thumb IP joint to compensate for weakness of the

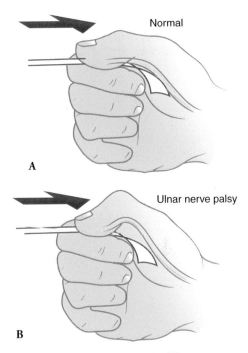

FIGURE 21-7 Normal pinch (**A**) and Froment sign (**B**).

first dorsal interosseous muscle adduction) (Fig. 21-7A and B), 2) Wartenburg sign (inability to adduct the small finger against the ring finger due to overpowering of the third palmar interosseous by the extensor digiti minimi) (Fig. 21-8), 3) an ulnar claw deformity (hyperextension of the metacarpophalangeal (MCP) joints with flexion of the proximal interphalangeal joints due to imbalance and overpowering of weak intrinsic muscles by the flexor digitorum profundus muscle) (Fig. 21-9).

Extrinsic radial nerve compression in the arm (Saturday night palsy) is much more common than intrinsic compression by a space-occupying lesion. The patient presents with wrist drop and loss of digital and thumb extension (Fig. 21-10A–B). The radial nerve can be compressed in the forearm (PIN) or at the wrist (radial sensory nerve). Compression of the PIN is known as posterior

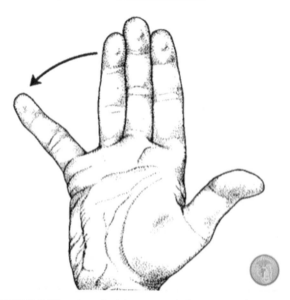

FIGURE 21-8 Wartenburg sign (ulnar nerve palsy).

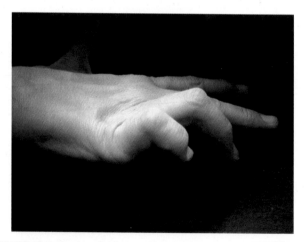

FIGURE 21-9 Clawing of the ulnar digits in low ulnar nerve palsy. (Picture courtesy of Ghazi Rayan MD).

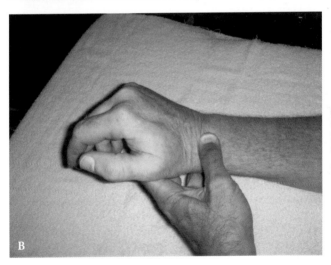

FIGURE 21-10 High radial nerve palsy with drop wrist and loss of active finger and thumb extension masked by the tenodesis effect caused by wrist flexion and by intact ulnar intrinsic function of proximal interphalangeal joint extension (**A**) and more manifest loss of active finger and thumb extension while the wrist is extended (**B**). (Pictures courtesy of Ghazi Rayan MD).

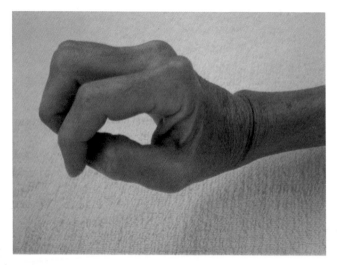

FIGURE 21-11 In PIN palsy when the patient is asked to extend the wrist, the wrist instead will radially deviate. Additionally there is loss of digital and thumb extension. (Picture courtesy of Ghazi Rayan MD).

interosseous nerve syndrome (Fig. 21-11), which preserves the extensor carpi radialis longus (patient maintains radial wrist extension) but causes a motor deficit in extensor carpi radialis brevis (loss of wrist extension) and extensor digitorum communis and extensor pollicis longus (loss of digital and thumb extensors). Another entity called radial tunnel syndrome is due to compression of the radial nerve before its bifurcation in the elbow and is characterized by mid-forearm pain without sensory or motor deficits. Wartenburg syndrome (or cheiralgia paresthetica) is compression of the radial sensory nerve between the brachioradialis and the extensor carpi radialis brevis muscles in the forearm due to repetitive pronation. All of these syndromes are managed initially with observation and modification of habits in using the hand for 3 to 6 months, followed by surgical decompression if symptoms persist.

Thoracic outlet syndrome is the compression of the brachial plexus that leads to paresthesias and weakness in the hand and upper extremity particularly in C8 and T1 lower trunk distribution. It can be of vascular or neurogenic nature. A supraclavicular or infraclavicular Tinel sign that produces paresthesias in the hand is indicative of nerve compression. Positive provocative maneuvers that aid in the diagnosis of thoracic outlet syndrome can produce vascular (diminished or absent radial pulse) or neurogenic (paresthesias) response. These include Roos test (reproduction of symptoms by holding hands overhead and pumping fists for 1 minute), costoclavicular maneuver (symptoms provoked by the exaggerated military maneuver of the shoulders), hyperabduction test (symptoms provoked with full shoulder abduction and external rotation), and Adson test (tilting chin upward and rotating head toward examiner). Treatment includes activity modifications and therapy for strengthening of the thoracic openers (levators, rhomboids, and upper trapezius muscles). Severe cases that do not respond to nonoperative treatment may benefit from cervical rib or first rib resection.

MISCELLANEOUS

Parsonage–Turner syndrome is a condition of unknown etiology but believed to be of viral origin and causes brachial neuritis. Initially there is acute, intense shoulder pain with an associated viral prodrome, followed by flaccid paralysis. A similar viral etiology has been described for some forms of AIN dysfunction. Both of these conditions are treated with observation.

CHAPTER 22

Musculotendinous System

FLEXOR TENDONS

Congenital anomalies that may affect the flexor musculotendinous structures include congenital absence of flexor muscles and tendons and cerebral palsy. Cerebral palsy is a non-progressive injury to the developing central nervous system that leads to hand and upper-limb dysfunction caused by muscle spasticity and contracture. Severe and untreated spasticity of the upper extremity in these children may result in deformities in the form of shoulder adduction, elbow flexion, forearm pronation, wrist flexion, digital flexion or swan neck deformity, and thumb in palm deformity (Fig. 22-1A–B).

When a volar skin laceration over the hand or wrist occurs a flexor tendon laceration must be ruled out. Early diagnosis of injuries to the digital flexor tendons determines the final outcome of digital motion. The flexor cascade of the fingers should be observed. In the normal digital flexor cascade each finger is slightly more flexed than the adjacent radial finger (Fig. 22-2). Hence the small finger is more flexed than the ring finger, which is more flexed than the middle finger, which is more flexed than the index finger. If a finger is "out of cascade," one or both of its flexor tendons most probably have been lacerated (Fig. 22-3).

The tenodesis test is a valuable physical examination test that aids in the diagnosis of flexor tendon injury. Due to the inherent muscle tone of the digital extrinsic flexors and extensors, passive wrist flexion and extension should lead to digital extension and flexion, respectively. If a lacerated finger does not demonstrate the tenodesis effect with passive wrist motion, an extrinsic tendon laceration should be suspected.

The key to examination of the individual flexor tendons is to remember that the flexor digitorum superficialis (FDS) tendons are capable of independent finger flexion, while the flexor digitorum profundus (FDP) tendons are not. Therefore, to isolate FDS function

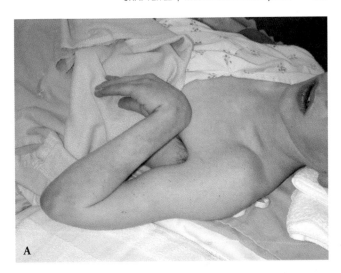

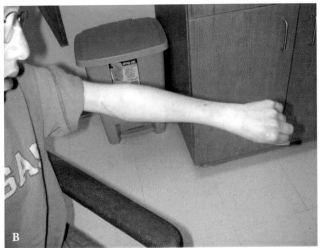

FIGURE 22-1 A patient with cerebral palsy and severe flexion contracture of the elbow and wrist due to long standing flexor muscle spasticity, before (**A**) and after wrist fusion and elbow flexion release (**B**). (Pictures are courtesy of Ghazi Rayan MD).

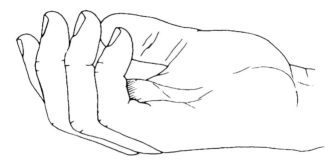

FIGURE 22-2 The normal flexor tendon cascade of the fingers.

the fingers other than the one in question are held in extension while the patient is instructed to actively flex the injured digit (Fig. 22-4). If the FDS tendon is intact, the patient should be able to actively flex the proximal interphalangeal (PIP) joint of the injured digit. The exception is the occasional interconnection between the FDS tendons of the ring and small fingers. When the small finger FDS is being tested the ring finger may need to be released and allowed to flex along with the small finger. The patient may have congenital hypoplasia or absence of the FDS to the small finger, which is frequently bilateral. As for all tendon examinations, FDS function should be checked against resistance. Occasionally, a

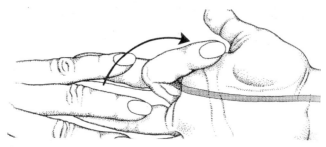

FIGURE 22-3 Testing the FDS is performed by asking the patient to flex the digit while holding the adjacent digits in extension to block the action of the flexor digitorum profundus.

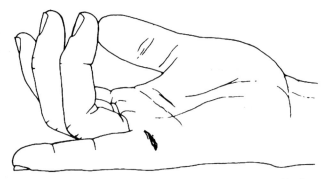

FIGURE 22-4 A finger "out of cascade" suggests that one or both of its flexor are severed.

tendon may be completely lacerated or avulsed with some retained function due to soft tissue attachments to the skeleton, such as its vinculum (blood supply). These alternate connections will not be sufficient to provide flexion power against resistance. Acute partial tendon lacerations are diagnosed by observing flexion against resistance with associated pain.

During examination of each finger's FDP tendon, the other fingers do not need to be restrained. The middle phalanx of the finger in question is held in extension and the patient is instructed to actively flex the injured distal interphalangeal (DIP) joint. If the FDP tendon is intact, this motion should be possible (Fig. 22-5). This needs to be checked against resistance to rule out partial tendon tears or the weak motion provided by the remaining non-tendinous soft tissue connections following a complete laceration.

The flexor pollicis longus (FPL) tendon is tested in a similar fashion to the FDP. The thumb's proximal phalanx is stabilized in extension and the patient is asked to actively flex the thumb interphalangeal (IP) joint (Fig. 22-6). IP joint flexion is checked against resistance.

In children with digital lacerations, tendon injuries should be suspected and ruled out. In young children, who may not be very cooperative with an examination, providing a toy to play with and

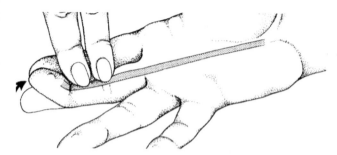

FIGURE 22-5 Testing of flexor digitorum profundus (FDP) is performed by blocking the PIP joint in full extension while having the patient flex the DIP joint.

observing for active flexion of the involved digital joints can be helpful. Children's wounds may need to be explored under anesthesia if the diagnosis is in question.

A common chronic source of tendon pathology is "stenosing tenosynovitis." In this condition the tendon may enlarge or the sheath that the tendon glides through becomes less compliant and narrower, leading to a constriction around the tendon, inhibiting motion. This is most common for the FDS tendons and FPL tendon, where the condition presents as a trigger digit, where the finger will "trigger," "get stuck," or even "lock." Digital motion will not be

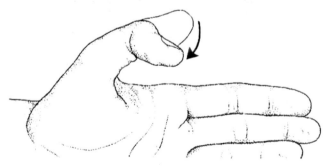

FIGURE 22-6 Testing of FPL is performed by blocking the thumb MP joint in extension while having the patient flex the IP joint.

smooth, but after full flexion there is a catch upon attempted extension. Conversely, the thumb IP joint may get "stuck" in extension and has difficulty flexing. This is often worse in the morning because of tissue edema and lower body temperature. There is often a tender nodule at the level of the A1 pulley of the flexor sheath, located over the volar metacarpophalangeal (MP) joint. In early cases triggering or catching may not be obvious and each patient presents with pain and tenderness over the A1 pulley associated with decreased active range of motion; passive range of motion is preserved.

Stenosing tenosynovitis may affect the flexor carpi radialis tendon. In these cases, the tendon is tender just proximal to the volar wrist crease and the patient's volar wrist pain is reproduced with resisted wrist flexion and full passive extension. The flexor carpi ulnaris tendon does not run in a sheath and is therefore not vulnerable to constrictive tenosynovitis. However, tendon degeneration, known as tendinosis or tendinopathy, may be associated with pisiform ligament complex syndrome. On physical examination, the flexor carpi ulnaris tendon will be tender proximal to the volar wrist crease and the patient's volar–ulnar sided wrist pain will be reproduced with resisted wrist flexion.

Infections of the flexor sheath or suppurative flexor tenosynovitis can be diagnosed by the four Kanavel signs (Chapter 19).

EXTENSOR TENDONS

Complete laceration of the digital extensor tendon over the DIP joint or the distal phalanx leads to "mallet finger" deformity and extensor lag of the joint. Similar injury and deformity can affect the thumb IP joint. In extensor lag the affected joint can be passively extended and is different from joint "flexion contracture," that is not passively correctable.

Injuries to the central slip over the PIP joint or the proximal phalanx lead to loss of active extension of the joint and later to a "boutonniere deformity." This deformity is characterized by flexion of the PIP and hyperextension of the DIP joint. In this condition, all of the digit's extensor power is shifted to the DIP joint by the lateral bands, leading to compensatory hyperextension of this joint. Because this deformity requires volar subluxation of the lateral bands to occur, it may not become manifest for 10–21 days following injury.

On examination, an acute central slip injury should be suspected if the patient is unable to attain PIP joint extension or is unable to maintain PIP joint extension against resistance. Three other tests for central slip integrity are the passive resistance, the Boyes DIP joint, and Elson tests. (i) With passive wrist and MP joint flexion the intact central slip will passively extend the PIP joint; failure for this to occur implies loss of central slip integrity. (ii) Inability of the patient to actively flex the DIP joint with the PIP joint held fully extended occurs when the central slip is disrupted, because the digit's extensor force is concentrated on the DIP joint. (iii) Elson test with the finger over a table edge and PIP joint flexed to 90 degrees,, the patient is asked to extend the PIP and DIP joints against resistance. This is possible normally but not when the central slip is injured.

Injuries to the digital extensor tendon over the MP joint or proximal to that may lead to an extensor lag at the MP joint. The index and small digits have more than one extrinsic extensor tendon. In partial and complete tendon lacerations the juncturae tendinea interconnections between the extensor digitorum communis (EDC) tendons allow active but weak MP joint extension. Therefore extension must be assessed against resistance. If MP joint extension cannot be maintained against resistance due to pain and/or weakness, an extensor tendon injury should be suspected.

The abductor pollicis longus tendon (first compartment) function is assessed by asking the patient to radially abduct the thumb, that is, "bring it away from the index finger" and palpating the taut tendon. Because the extensor pollicis longus (EPL) extends both the thumb MP and IP joints it is difficult to assess for isolated extensor pollicis brevis laceration. An extensor lag of the thumb MP joint or pain with resisted MP joint extension is suggestive of extensor pollicis brevis tendon injury.

The extensor carpi radialis brevis and extensor carpi radialis longus tendons (second compartment) are assessed by asking the patient to extend and radially deviate the wrist while making a fist. Weakness of extension against resistance suggests injury to extensor carpi radialis brevis and against radial deviation suggests injury to extensor carpi radialis longus tendon.

The EPL tendon (third compartment) is the only tendon that allows retropulsion of the thumb (extend it dorsal to the plane of the palm). The thumb intrinsic muscles can cause weak IP joint extension. Therefore to assess EPL tendon integrity, it is not enough to visualize active IP joint extension. The patient is seated with both hands flat on a table, then asked to lift up the thumbs off the table. In case of EPL laceration, the patient will not be able to raise the thumb off the resting surface.

The EDC tendons (fourth compartment) can be evaluated by having the patient extend the fingers' MP joints against resistance with the wrist extended (Fig. 22-7). The extensor indicis proprius can be evaluated by having the patient extend the index finger

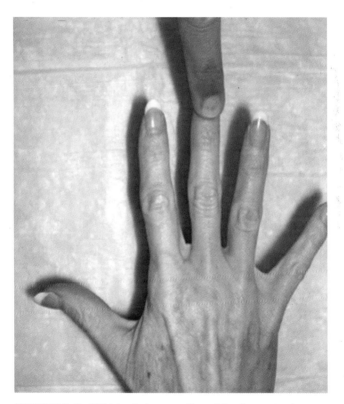

FIGURE 22-7 The EDC integrity is assessed by resistive finger extension.

against resistance with the other digits flexed. In children, or noncooperative patients, the tenodesis test is again helpful where passive flexion of the wrist will cause the fingers and thumb to extend if the EDC and EPL tendons are intact; this does not occur if the extensor tendon is severed.

The extensor digiti minimi tendon (fifth compartment) can be evaluated by having the patient extend the small finger with the other digits flexed.

The extensor carpi ulnaris (ECU) tendon (sixth compartment) can be evaluated by having the patient extend and ulnar deviate the wrist against resistance while palpating the taut tendon.

Any of the six extensor tendon compartments of the wrist may be affected by stenosing tenosynovitis. Stenosing tenosynovitis of the first dorsal compartment is known as DeQuervain tenosynovitis. Patients with this condition exhibit pain and sometimes swelling over the first dorsal compartment, located on the radial side of the wrist. Finkelstein in 1930 described a maneuver to diagnose DeQuervain tendonitis. In the Finkelstein test (Fig. 22-8A–B) the thumb metacarpal is passively adducted or the patient tucks their thumb in their palm, makes a fist, and gently ulnar deviates their wrist. Reproduction of the patient's pain constitutes a positive test.

Stenosing tenosynovitis of the second dorsal compartment is known as intersection syndrome. This name is a misnomer; the pathology is similar to other stenosing tenosynovitis and not due to friction between tendons, as originally believed. The tendons of the first and second compartments run in separate sheaths and are not in contact. This condition is due to repetitive wrist extension, such as during raking leaves, shoveling, gardening, and occasionally athletic activities. The patient has pain, tenderness, and swelling located dorsal and 4–8 cm proximal to the radial styloid, well proximal to the area of tenderness for DeQuervain disease. Pain is reproduced by resisted wrist extension and often by forced wrist flexion. Palpable crepitus or squeaking may be present.

Stenosing tenosynovitis of the third, fourth, and fifth compartments may also occur but is uncommon. Pain, tenderness, and often swelling occur over the involved compartments. Pain is reproduced by resisted extension of the EPL tendon (third compartment), EDC tendons (fourth compartments), or the small finger, the extensor digiti minimi tendon.

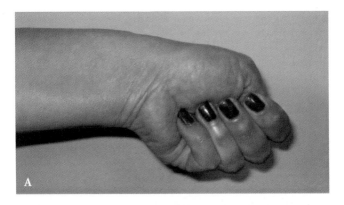

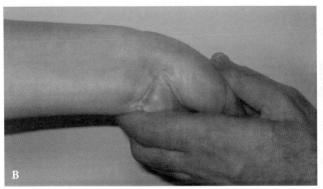

FIGURE 22-8 Finkelstein test is performed by having the patient grasp their thumb with their fingers then gently move their wrist into ulnar deviation (**A**). An alternative is passively adduct the patients thumb metacarpal (**B**). Reproduction of the patient's pain constitutes a positive test and confirms the diagnosis of DeQuervain disease.

Stenosing tenosynovitis of the sixth compartment leads to pain, tenderness, and often swelling over the ECU tendon. Pain is provoked with resisted wrist extension and ulnar deviation. In addition, the sixth compartment ECU sub-sheath may become attenuated, leading to ulnar subluxation of the ECU tendon. This can lead to a painful snapping on the ulnar side of the wrist with ulnar deviation and supination. With the elbow resting on an examination table and the forearm supinated, the ECU tendon may sublux if the patient ulnar deviates the wrist against resistance. In severe cases, the ECU may be manually displaced ulnarly by the examiner, recreating the patient's symptoms.

INTRINSIC TENDONS

The intrinsic muscles flex the MP joint and extend the PIP and DIP joints. They also abduct and adduct the fingers. Intrinsic function can be evaluated by having the patient abduct the digits against resistance; ulnar nerve palsy with paralysis of intrinsic muscles will lead to weakness of digital abduction. The patient's ability to hold their fingers in the "intrinsic plus" position, of MP joint flexion with PIP and DIP joint extension, can also be compromised and the fingers assume the "intrinsic minus" position of MP joint hyperextension and PIP and DIP joint flexion. This is also known as "clawing" and usually most pronounced in the ring and small fingers, because the lumbrical muscles to the index and middle fingers are innervated by the median nerve.

The intrinsic system may also become contracted or tight from post-traumatic scarring, spasticity due to stroke or upper motor neuron injury, or inflammatory diseases, such as rheumatoid arthritis. When this occurs, the fingers may be held in the posture with the least stretch on the intrinsic muscles, that is, MP joint flexion and PIP joint extension. The patient cannot extend the MP joint while flexing the PIP and DIP joints. This leads to difficulty with "large object grasp," such as holding a glass. The patient perceives weakness of grip and inability to close their hand around the object (because the fingers cannot flex any more, so no power can be generated). However, the patient is able to easily make a fist, which involves MP joint flexion. MP joint flexion relaxes the intrinsic muscles, allowing PIP and DIP joint flexion to occur.

The Bunnell intrinsic tightness test helps to diagnose intrinsic tightness (Fig. 22-9). The test is performed by holding the finger MP joint extended by the examiner. If passive PIP joint flexion is not possible, then it is because of the presence of either PIP joint contracture or intrinsic muscles tightness. If flexing the MP joint does not allow the PIP joint to flex, then the lack of motion is due

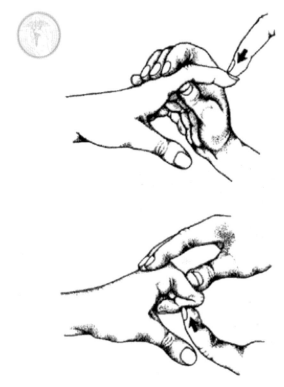

FIGURE 22-9 The Bunnell intrinsic tightness test: PIP joint flexion is less with the MP joint extended than with the MP joint flexed.

to joint contracture. However, if PIP joint flexion is possible only during MP joint flexion (but not with it extended), then it confirms the diagnosis of intrinsic tightness.

Extrinsic tightness can affect extensor (EDC) or flexor (FDS and FDP) muscles. In extrinsic extensor contracture the patient cannot make a fist and flex the digital joints while the wrist is flexed. Flexing the digital joints is easier with the wrist is flexed. A variant of this test is the need to extend the MP joint in order to flex the PIP and DIP joints. If the degree of PIP joint flexion is independent of MP joint position, then a contracture of the PIP joint itself exists. In extrinsic flexor muscle contracture the reverse is true where passive digital extension is not possible while the wrist is extended but becomes easier with wrist flexion.

TREATMENT

Closed or open complete flexor tendon injury should be treated by surgical repair or reconstruction. Extensor tendon lacerations should be repaired. For the terminal extensor tendon, it is appropriate that closed injuries are treated closed, while open injuries are treated open, that is, surgically. Most closed sagittal band injuries with EDC tendon subluxation can be treated nonoperativly but those with chronic painful dislocation usually require surgical reconstruction (see Chapter 23).

Intrinsic spasticity is initially treated nonoperatively by stretching and splinting under the direction of a hand therapist. Loss of hand function due to intrinsic muscle paralysis is treated by tendon transfers where another tendon is attached to the intrinsic tendons to restore function.

Infections of the flexor sheath should be treated emergently. If recognized within the first 24–48 hours, they can be treated with hospitalization and intravenous antibiotics. If the infection resolves rapidly, then surgical irrigation and debridement will usually not be necessary. If seen after 48 hours following the onset of the infection, or if the infection fails to rapidly respond to nonoperative measures, then surgical irrigation and debridement is indicated (see Chapter 19).

CHAPTER 23

Retinacular System

Examination of the retinacular supports of the hand and wrist is used to determine their normal and abnormal function and integrity. Abnormal function of the retinacular system components is sometimes evident at rest (e.g., Boutonnière deformity) and occasionally with motion (e.g., flexor tendon bowstringing and sagittal band dislocation).

FLEXOR RETINACULAR COMPLEX OF THE WRIST

The transverse carpal ligament (TCL) restrains the flexor tendons from volar migration, especially during simultaneous wrist and digital flexion. Releasing the TCL is a standard procedure for treating carpal tunnel syndrome. This does not usually have any adverse clinical effect and does not cause tendinous instability. However, under certain circumstances, such as excising rather than incising the TCL, flexor tendinous instability may develop. Failure of the TCL to heal after a severe injury might result in volar subluxation of the flexor tendons. Although uncommon, this condition is diagnosed by palpating a snap when the flexor tendons *jump* volar and ulnar to the hook of the hamate. During powerful grasp the wrist tends to deviate ulnarward. The ulnar direction of pull by the flexors during simultaneous wrist and digital flexion contributes to this phenomenon when the TCL is incompetent. Examination of the proximal or the distal edge of the TCL may reveal the presence of a soft tissue *mass* due to associated tenosynovitis. The distal retinacular edge is more distinct to palpation than the proximal edge. The characteristics of the mass, if present, should be determined by inspection and palpation as in evaluating any other hand tumor. In particular the following should be observed: adherence, consistency, color, size, shape, surface, turgor, and tenderness. Generally, the mass effect of tenosynovitis, regardless of cause, will move with digital flexion and extension.

EXTENSOR RETINACULUM OF THE WRIST

The six extensor compartments of the wrist deep to the retinaculum can be individually palpated. Tenderness may be elicited in the first, third, fifth, or sixth compartments due to tendinopathy (Chapter 22). Each of the compartments is located within a tightly confined space. As such, changes in compartments shape or increase in their contents size can alter the biomechanics and blood flow to tendons and thus contribute to tendinopathy. The examiner should be able to identify the location of the compartments using underlying bony anatomy. The first dorsal compartment is in proximity to the radial styloid and the sixth to the ulnar styloid. Of importance also is palpating Lister tubercle (third compartment) and the dorsal aspect of the distal radioulnar joint (fifth compartment). Pathology of these compartments, from direct soft-tissue injury, tendon swelling, or bony irregularity (from fracture or arthritis), can result in tendon irritation, pain, and even attrition and rupture.

FLEXOR PULLEY SYSTEM

The flexor tendons move beneath the flexor pulleys a distance equal to the joint circumference traveled. For the purpose of understanding the distance traveled, the tendons should be considered inelastic. It is important to recall that the flexor digitorum superficialis (FDS) tendon moves the proximal interphalangeal (PIP) joint and thus does not need to move as far as the flexor digitorum profundus tendon during full finger flexion. The total distance either flexor tendons move within the sheath is approximately 4 cm in an average-sized hand. However, the same tendon that moves 4 cm in the finger must move an additional 4 cm in the palm and wrist to allow full finger and concomitant wrist motion. In conjunction with the unobstructed excursion, the pulley system must be smooth and enable unimpeded differential motion of the FDS and flexor digitorum profundus tendons to allow distal interphalangeal

(DIP) joint extension at the same time that full PIP joint flexion is employed.

The most common pathology that affects this system of pulleys is tenosynovitis, which may cause triggering as seen in *trigger finger*. Catching of the enlarged FDS tendon will be often at proximal edge of the A1 pulley and the trigger phenomena is actually the tendon tucking back into the sheath after it has bunched up in the palm.

Tendon sheath rupture can occur in the presence of great forces generated from tendons on the pulleys. Usually this occurs among healthy young adults who apply a heavy and often sudden load to the finger. It may complicate flexor tendon surgery if the important pulleys were not repaired (Fig. 23-1). This frequently presents as pain along the sheath due to rupture of the A2 pulley among rock climbers. The presentation is classic in that the injury occurred suddenly, usually with a *pop* and subsequent onset of swelling and perhaps bowstringing. The flexion strength will be reduced and magnetic resonance imaging (MRI) will reveal the tendon(s) to be displaced anteriorly away from the P1.

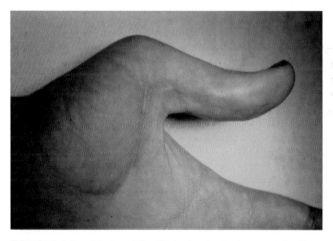

FIGURE 23-1 Bowstringing of the FPL tendon due to damage of the flexor pulley system of the thumb. (Picture courtesy of Ghazi Rayan MD).

RETINACULAR ASSEMBLY OF THE EXTENSOR MECHANISM

Sagittal Band

As noted in the anatomy section, the sagittal band guides the extensor digitorum communis (EDC) tendon during metacarpophalangeal (MP) joint flexion. Sagittal band injury may be associated with swelling and pain in the area adjacent to the metacarpal head. The patient may have a history of direct injury as laceration or indirect trauma such as repetitive gripping or flipping the finger. Sagittal band injury can be classified into type I, mild without EDC instability, type II, moderate with subluxation, and type III, severe with dislocation of the EDC (Fig. 23-2). Complete rupture of the radial sagittal band leads to ulnar dislocation of the EDC away from the metacarpal head. A visible "snap" and instability of the extensor tendons into the valley of the intermetacarpal space will occur. There are two tests for sagittal band injuries: (i) resistive digital extension abduction test for type I injury which provokes pain (Fig. 23-3) and (ii) patients with type III injury will be able to maintain a passively extended MP joint, but will not be able to actively extend the MP joint from a flexed position (Fig. 23-4).

Complete attenuation with type III sagittal band injury is encountered in rheumatoid arthritis. The examiner needs to asses the integrity of the collateral ligaments and rule out their injury. This can best be done with MP joint flexion to about 70 degrees and applying stress in radial and ulnar directions. In both directions the joint should be stable if the ligaments are intact. Pain caused by this maneuver suggests partial injury to the collateral ligament. Direct trauma as in boxing may be associated with sagittal band and dorsal capsular tear of the MP joint.

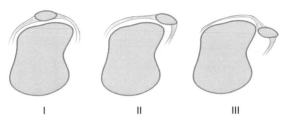

FIGURE 23-2 The three types of sagittal band injuries. (Rayan G and Murray D 1994).

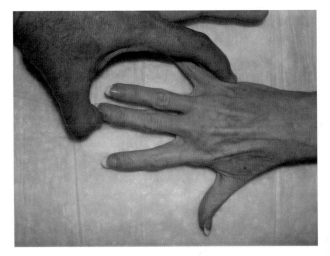

FIGURE 23-3 Test for sagittal band injury especially for type I. Resistive finger abduction provokes pain in the area adjacent to the MP joint.

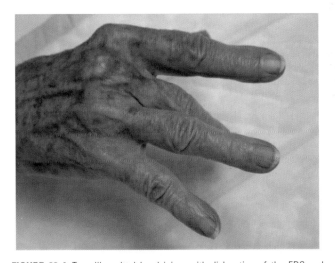

FIGURE 23-4 Type III sagittal band injury with dislocation of the EDC and inability to actively extend the MP joint. (Pictures courtesy of Ghazi Rayan MD).

Triangular and Transverse Retinacular Ligaments

Any patient who sustains a direct end-on (stave) injury to the fingertip is at risk for rupturing the central slip, which can be followed by attenuation of the triangular ligament. Similarly, injury to the palmar plate may occur with the development of swan neck deformity. Examining a swollen PIP joint should raise suspicion for central slip rupture and incipient *boutonnière* "button hole" deformity that will follow. This injury will frequently impact adjacent DIP joint, lateral bands, triangular ligament, and transverse retinacular ligament. Assuming an X-ray rules out fractures, the next step is to determine whether the patient can maintain the PIP joint in full extension both actively and against resistance. Weakness of PIP joint extension against resistance is suggestive of central slip injury. When boutonnière deformity develops (Fig. 23-5) the lateral bands migrate volar to the axis of joint motion and the triangular ligament becomes

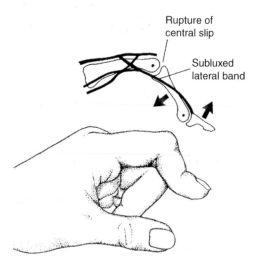

Rupture of
central slip

Subluxed
lateral band

FIGURE 23-5 Central slip injury over the PIP joint will lead to loss of active extension of the joint and eventually to a "boutonnière deformity" due to volar migration of the lateral bands.

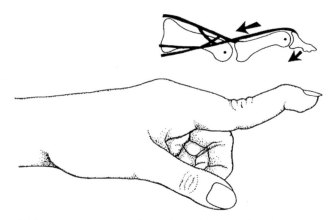

FIGURE 23-6 In swan neck deformity there is hyperextension of the PIP joint and dorsal migration of the lateral bands.

attenuated and at the same time the transverse retinacular ligament will shorten and contract. Conversely when swan neck deformity of the PIP joint develops (Fig. 23-6) the opposite occurs where the lateral bands migrate dorsal, the triangular ligament becomes shortened, and at the same time the transverse retinacular ligament will elongate and attenuate.

Understanding the relationships of these deformities with the pathology inflicted upon the various retaining ligaments of the extensor mechanism is imperative for their definitive treatment.

DEEP RETINACULAR STRUCTURES OF THE HAND

The clinical relevance of these anatomical structures lies in the damage that can be inflicted on the interpalmar plate ligament during crushing injuries or lacerations and in Dupuytren disease that may involve the septa of Legueu and Juvara leading to the development of vertical cord in the palm. The transverse ligament of the palmr aponeurosis (TLPA) may be affected in Dupuytren disease because of its attachment in the septa of Legueu and Juvara. Involvement of these anatomical structures can be confirmed only during surgery.

RETAINING LIGAMENTS OF THE SKIN

The clinical relevance of Cleland and Grayson ligaments is seen primarily in the course of examination and treatment of Dupuytren disease or during surgery for correcting swan neck deformity and post-traumatic PIP joint contracture. Dupuytren disease can involve these tissues and, as such, act as a restraint to the extension of the PIP and rarely the DIP joints (see Chapter 18).

CHAPTER 24

Syndesmotic System

WRIST

Ligament injuries of the wrist may be acute and usually develop after substantial trauma, such as a fall on the outstretched hand and wrist, or they may be chronic from repetitive use where the patient may not recall a specific traumatic event. In both scenarios, the patient presents with a painful wrist. The diagnosis of a major carpal derangement in both the acute and chronic settings can be made with a careful history, a thorough wrist examination, and by obtaining appropriate X-rays and other imaging studies.

Clinical Examination

Physical examination is preceded by a thorough history, which includes the mechanism of injury. Details about the exact location of pain in the wrist, aggravating and relieving factors, and prior treatments are important to obtain. Other than in open dislocations, the external appearance of most wrist instabilities may be subtle. Frequently, carpal instabilities are missed due to the lack of an obvious clinical deformity. Swelling is generally mild or moderate and may be present only in the acute injury setting such as skin abrasions, contusions, or ecchymotic areas.

In acute ligament injuries, wrist range of motion is limited by pain, however, wrist motion may be almost normal in chronic cases. Localizing the area of wrist tenderness is imperative for identifying the injured structure and making the precise diagnosis. The most common areas of specific tenderness are the anatomical snuffbox, scapholunate (SL) joint (just distal and ulnar to Lister's tubercle), the LT joint (2 cm distal to the ulnar head), and at the level of the triangular fibrocartilage complex (TFCC) (immediately distal to the ulnar head). In subacute and chronic cases, applying passive wrist motion is valuable not only in detecting abnormal motion and inciting crepitus but also in reproducing pain. Grip strength may be weakened by actual loss of muscle strength from disuse or caused by pain. Specific stress tests for these individual ligament injuries are described later. At least 2 X-ray views of the wrist should be obtained, a true posteroanterior (PA) and lateral views. Often, having a third view will help in better defining anatomy. If a diagnosis is still uncertain, other X-rays such as a 10-degree pronated view may allow more precise identification of a scapholunate gap and may be suggestive of scapholunate interosseous ligament (SLIL) injury.

Perilunate Instability

Acute perilunate instabilities are present in a predictable pattern of progression beginning with SLIL injury and evolving to end-stage carpal lunate dislocates from the distal radius articular surface. There may be distortion of the carpal tunnel anatomy, which may compress the median nerve causing acute neuropathy. Acute instability may only involve the wrist ligaments (lesser arc injury) or be combined with fractures (greater arc injury). The lesser arc pattern begins with force initiation at the SLIL and progresses through the capitolunate joint and exits out through the lunotriquetral interosseous ligament (LTIL). A greater arc injury initiates at the radial side of the wrist with a scaphoid or radial styloid fracture and progresses through the capitolunate joint and exits through the triquetrum (Fig. 24-1).

In acute carpal ligament injuries and perilunate dislocations, the lateral X-ray is critical in making the correct diagnosis. Radiographic findings are most dramatic in carpal dislocations. The head of the capitate should fit in the center of the distal lunate cup, which should then align with the shaft and center of the articular surface of the radius. A substantial carpal ligament injury is suggested by disruption of this linkage. If the capitate head no longer articulates with the center of the lunate cup and is located dorsal to the lunate, this confirms the diagnosis of perilunate dislocation (Fig. 24-2). If the capitate head is articulating with the distal radius and the lunate is displaced, volar, to the articular surface of the distal radius, this is synonymous with a lunate dislocation (Fig. 24-3). The PA X-ray view may be helpful in diagnosing associated fractures of the scaphoid, distal radius, or other carpal bones.

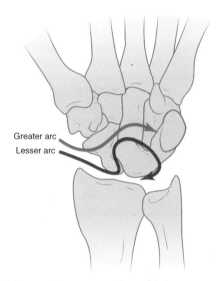

Greater arc
Lesser arc

FIGURE 24-1 Lesser and greater arc perilunate injuries.

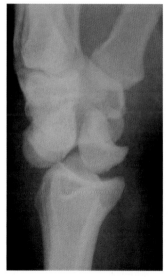

FIGURE 24-2 A lateral X-ray view of perilunate dislocation. The carpus dislocates around the intact lunate. The head of the capitate is dorsal to the lunate.

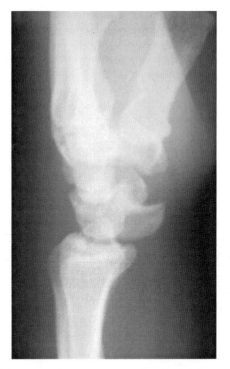

FIGURE 24-3 Lunate dislocation. In advanced stage of perilunate injury, the carpus is reduced and pushes the lunate volar to the radius out of the lunate fossa of the distal radius, which becomes occupied by the capitate.

Scapholunate Interosseous Ligament Injury

Injuries to the SLIL are a common source of wrist pain and represent the most common form of wrist instability. This presents as tenderness at the SL interval located in the soft spot 1 cm distal to Lister's tubercle and in the snuffbox. Pain will usually be elicited with forced wrist extension. In established cases, the scaphoid shift test may be positive (Fig. 24-4). This test is performed by holding the wrist in slight flexion while moving from ulnar into radial deviation. During this maneuver, the thumb of the examiner places dorsal pressure on the scaphoid tubercle, located just proximal-ulnar to the

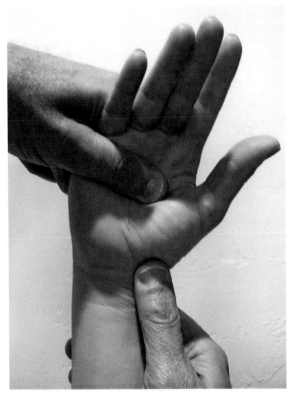

FIGURE 24-4 Scaphoid shift test.

trapeziometacarpal (TM) joint and just distal-radial to the most distal visible portion of the flexor carpi radialis tendon. This prevents the scaphoid from moving in concert with the lunate when the SLIL is injured. This maneuver is considered positive if it reproduces a symptomatic pop in the wrist that is not present on the contralateral wrist, or if it elicits dorsal wrist pain over the SL interval. In acute carpal injuries that are not associated with dislocation, the X-ray findings may not be always diagnostic. Attention is given to the distance between the scaphoid and lunate. If the space between

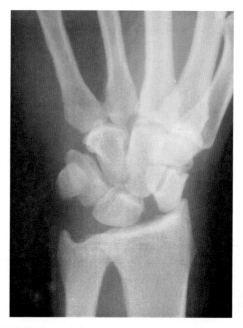

FIGURE 24-5 Static scapholunate interosseous ligament (SLIL) injury due to complete rupture of the ligament with wide SL gap.

these two bones is greater than 4 to 5 mm, this suggests complete SLIL rupture (Fig. 24-5). There is some variability in the SL distance and obtaining a comparison view of the opposite wrist may provide clarification. Widening of scapholunate distance >1 to 2 mm from the opposite wrist may indicate instability and partial SLIL injury. Further radiographic studies such as AP ulnar deviation and "clenched fist" views may further widen the SL space.

In carpal ligament injuries, measurement of carpal angles on the lateral X-ray view may be helpful for diagnosis (Fig. 24-6). It is important to identify the dorsal and volar lips of the lunate, the long axis of the scaphoid and capitate, and the center of the distal radius. The long axis of the capitate, lunate, and radial shaft should be colinear. In a SLIL injury, the lunate extends and the capitate shifts dorsal, a condition also termed dorsal intercalated segment

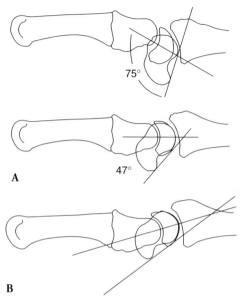

FIGURE 24-6 A scapholunate angle of 75 degrees is an indication of torn SL ligament **(A)**. The normal SL angle is approximately 47 degrees (range 30–60 degrees). A scapholunate angle of 15 degrees **(B)** is an indication for a tear in the LT ligament. (Figure is a combination of pages 87 & 88 from Seiler JG III. *Essentials of Hand Surgery.* Philadelphia: Lippincott Williams & Wilkins; 2002).

instability (DISI) pattern. The scapholunate angle normally is 45 degrees (range 30 to 60 degrees); this angle also increases outside the normal range in DISI.

In some cases, X-rays may be normal because secondary restraints may limit the altered motion. Carpal instability is classified into dynamic or static instability. In dynamic instability, the X-rays may be normal and the instability may manifest only when load is placed across the wrist. In static carpal instability, the abnormal carpal relationships are apparent on standard X-rays (Fig. 24-5). Wrist arthroscopy can provide definitive evidence of ligament abnormalities along with assessment of coexisting pathology in the wrist.

Lunotriquetral Interosseous Ligament Injury

The LTIL is a less common source of wrist pain. LTIL injury is associated with tenderness in the LT articulation. The LT articulation lies in the soft spot ulnar and slightly proximal to the SL articulation. The shear and shuck tests may be helpful in establishing the diagnosis. In the shuck test, the lunate is grasped between the thumb and index finger of one hand, and the triquetrum and pisiform (which lies immediately volar to the triquetrum) is grasped between the thumb and index finger of the other hand. The two bones are then moved dorsally and volarly against each other in pronation, neutral rotation, and supination. In the shear test, the examiner's thumb applies dorsally directed pressure against the volar pisiform while the index finger applies a volar pressure against the dorsal lunate. The wrist is then radially and ulnarly deviated. Either of these tests is considered positive when the patient's dorsoulnar wrist pain is reproduced by these maneuvers.

There are minimal findings on X-ray for LTIL injuries. If the ligament between the lunate and triquetrum is ruptured, the lunate may palmar flex. Loss of the LT ligament may have no effect on the scapholunate angle or it may be less than 30 degrees (Fig. 24-6B).

Midcarpal Instability

Ligament injury may affect those, which span the proximal and distal carpal rows. Midcarpal ligament injuries are either acute or chronic. These ligaments ensure a smooth transition of the proximal carpal row as it moves from flexion to extension when the wrist deviates ulnarly. Patients with midcarpal instability typically present with a painful audible "clunk" as the wrist is brought from radial to ulnar deviation. The "clunk" occurs as the wrist snaps from a flexed to an extended posture instead of the normal smooth transition. Standard wrist X-rays are normal or may show a volar intercalated segment instability (VISI) pattern where the entire proximal carpal row appears flexed. This form of instability can best be demonstrated by video motion fluoroscopy ("cine" views). Conditions associated with ligament laxity can predispose to midcarpal instability including collagen disorders such as Ehlers–Danlos syndrome. A distal radius fracture, which has a significant dorsal angulation malunion, can also lead to instability called extrinsic midcarpal instability.

Table 24-1	Triangular Fibrocartilage Complex (TFCC) Abnormalities

Class 1: Traumatic

A. Central perforation

B. Ulnar avulsion (with or without ulnar styloid fracture)

C. Distal avulsion

D. Radial avulsion (with or without sigmoid notch fracture)

Class 2: Degenerative (ulnocarpal abutment syndrome)

A. TFCC wear

B. TFCC wear
+ Lunate and/or ulnar chondromalacia

C. TFCC perforation
+ Lunate and/or ulnar chondromalacia

D. TFCC perforation
+ Lunate and/or ulnar chondromalacia
+ L-T ligament perforation

E. TFCC perforation
+ Lunate and/or ulnar chondromalacia
+ L-T ligament perforation
+ Ulnocarpal arthritis

Triangular Fibrocartilage Complex

TFCC injuries can be either acute or chronic and classified (Palmer) into two main types, traumatic and degenerative (Table 24-1). The diagnosis is established by tenderness over the dorsal or volar aspect of the TFCC. Axial load and ulnar deviation of the wrist can also be used as a provocative maneuver to elicit pain and mechanical catching. X-rays are usually normal for TFCC tears. Arthrograms and magnetic resonance imaging can confirm the diagnosis.

An untreated chronic wrist ligament injury will lead to the development of a predictable pattern of wrist osteoarthritis. The most common pattern is caused by scapholunate instability and called scapholunate advanced collapse or SLAC wrist. Arthritic changes first occur at the radioscaphoid joint, as the normally congruous surfaces of the scaphoid and radius become incongruous. This progresses to

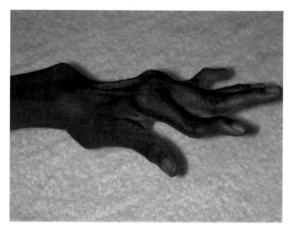

FIGURE 24-7 Rheumatoid arthritis of the wrist with distal radioulnar joint (DRUJ) dislocation and swan neck deformities of the proximal interphalangeal (PIP) joints. (Picture courtesy of Ghazi Rayan MD).

similar changes at the scaphocapitate joint followed by the capitolunate joint years later. Eventually, after many years, all articulations of the wrist joint may be affected with osteoarthritis.

Rheumatoid arthritis (RA) affects the wrist in a different manner. As inflammatory synovitis from this disease progressively weakens the carpal ligaments, the wrist may translate ulnarward along the distal radius inclination. This is accompanied by radial deviation deformity of the radiocarpal joint. This instability contributes to ulnar drift of the metacapophalangeal (MP) joints. Another common area affected by RA is the TFCC and distal radioulnar joint dislocation. As the inflammatory synovitis disrupts the TFCC attachment at the base of the ulnar styloid, the distal ulna appears to migrate dorsal, but actually, it is the volar subluxation of the radius that contributes to this finding (Fig. 24-7).

HAND

There are myriad of arthritic conditions that may affect the hand, the most common of which are osteoarthritis and rheumatoid arthritis. Posttraumatic arthritis develops in response to intra-articular fractures or chronic ligamentous injury and joint instability. Osteoarthritic joints are often enlarged and tender. Osteophytes or localized bony enlargements of the distal interphalangeal (DIP) joints are called "Heberden's nodules." Similar changes of the proximal interphalangeal (PIP) joints are called "Bouchard's nodules." Arthritic joints may have crepitus, or grinding, of the joints with motion. Subluxation may be present, but it is usually less painful than subluxation caused by an acute injury.

The TM joint of the thumb is the most frequently affected joint in the hand by osteoarthritis. Pain is referred to the base of the thumb and experienced during pinching and gripping, such as when writing, turning a key, opening a jar, holding a book, and other common activities of daily living. Arthritis of the TM joint is associated with dorsoradial subluxation of the first metacarpal against the trapezium. This can be observed as a dorsal step-off of the TM joint, known as the "shoulder sign." Symptomatic TM joints are often tender over the volar base of the first metacarpal at the proximal aspect of the thenar muscle mass. Provocative tests for the TM joint disease include the abduction test (where the hand is held stable and the thumb firmly abducted away from it), the adduction test (where the hand is held stable and the thumb firmly adducted into it), and the grind test (where the wrist is held stable and the first metacarpal compressed against the trapezium and firmly rotated).

In RA, there is associated attenuation or rupture of joint ligaments with resultant instability such as swan neck deformity of the PIP joints (Fig. 24-7), ulnar drift deformity of the MP joints (Fig. 24-8), or dislocation.

Traumatic ligament injuries in general including those of digital joints can be classified into three types of increasing severity. Type I is mild in the form of a simple sprain, Type II is moderate in the form of partial rupture or substantial elongation, and Type III represents a complete ligament tear, which may or may not be associated with joint dislocation. Acute traumatic ligament injuries of the digital joints that present in the emergency room are often in the form of joint dislocations. Digital joint dislocations are classified into simple or complex. Simple dislocations can be easily reduced by manipulation and do not need surgery. Complex dislocations cannot be reduced by closed methods because there is usually tissue entrapment that is blocking reduction.

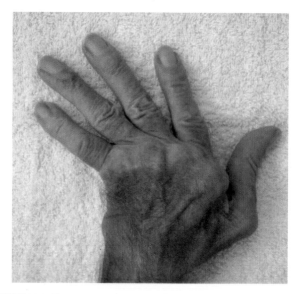

FIGURE 24-8 Rheumatoid arthritis of the hand with ulnar drift deformity of the MP joints. (Picture courtesy of Ghazi Rayan MD).

Ligament injuries in the hand may affect any digital joint including TM, MP, PIP, or DIP joint.

The most frequently affected joints with ligament injuries are the MP and PIP joints.

Metacarpophalangeal Joint

The ulnar collateral ligament of the thumb MP joint is the most frequently injured ligament in the hand. The patient presents with swelling and tenderness along the ulnar aspect of the thumb MP joint. Instability in case of type III ligament injury can be confirmed with a stress test (Fig. 24-9). X-rays, including stress views, may be helpful in making the diagnosis by demonstrating excessive angulation. A number of thumb ulnar collateral ligament injuries are associated with a small bone avulsion from the ulnar base of the proximal phalanx. A "Stenner lesion" occurs when the ulnar

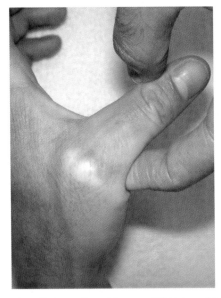

FIGURE 24-9 Type III ulnar collateral ligament (UCL) injury of the thumb MP joint is confirmed with a stress test. (Picture courtesy of Ghazi Rayan MD).

collateral ligament becomes detached from the base of the proximal phalanx and is folded back and entrapped superficial to the adductor aponeurosis. These often require surgical treatment.

In the fingers, complex dislocations occur most frequently in the MP joint of the index finger when the volar plate or another anatomic structure is interposed between metacarpal head and proximal phalanx base. Surgery is indicated to remove interposed tissue from the joint and facilitate reduction. The dorsal capsule of the MP joint is typically thin and weak. Radial collateral ligament injuries are more common than ulnar. Radial and ulnar collateral ligament injuries result from a lateral deviation of the finger, causing rupture in midsubstance or avulsion from bone. Midsubstance ruptures are less common. The ligaments of the index and small fingers, being border digits, are more commonly injured. Diagnosis is made by localized tenderness along the radial or ulnar margin of the joint.

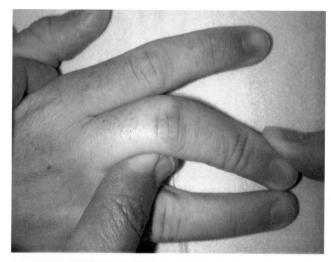

FIGURE 24-10 Type III radial collateral ligament (RCL) injury of the middle finger proximal interphalangeal (PIP) joint is confirmed with a stress test. (Picture courtesy of Ghazi Rayan MD).

Proximal Interphalangeal Joint

These may present as acute or chronic injuries. Type II ligament injuries can be difficult to diagnose. The patient presents with swelling and tenderness along the lateral aspect of the PIP joint. A stress X-ray view can be helpful in confirming the diagnosis (Fig. 24-10). When there is 20 degrees of angulation or difference with the contralateral normal side, this suggests Type II ligament injury. Greater than 30 degrees of lateral deviation with a stress test of the joint without endpoint suggests the diagnosis is of a complete ligament rupture. Using local anesthetic allows more accurate clinical assessment of joint instability during a stress test and for radiographic stress test examination. Type III acute injuries of the PIP joint are easy to diagnose, as these present in the form of dislocation that is easily seen on X-ray most often dorsal (Fig. 24-11) or lateral and less often palmar. Palmar dislocations tend to be complex and associated with less favorable treatment outcome and more complications than dorsal dislocation.

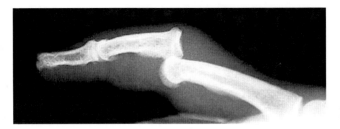

FIGURE 24-11 Radiographic appearance of dorsal proximal interphalangeal (PIP) joint dislocation.

Both MP and especially PIP joints can develop stiffness and joint contracture after ligament injury. Scarring of the ligaments with contracture often occurs after trauma or after prolonged digit immobilization, especially with the ligament in a shortened position. The latter affects the MP joint when immobilized in extension or neutral position rather than intrinsic plus position (flexion at the MP and extension of the PIP joint). The intrinsic plus posture maintains the collateral ligaments in their elongated position preventing their contracture. Scar tissue in the ligaments, especially those of the MP joint, may develop in response to unresolved edema of the dorsum of the hand. At the PIP joint, if the volar plate does not glide distally with extension, a flexion contracture may result. The proximal portion of the volar plate may form thick checkrein ligaments on the distal volar aspect of the P1 that limits gliding and contributes to PIP flexion contracture. Arthritis is initially treated nonoperatively with injections, nonsteroidal anti-inflammatory medications, and often by splint immobilization and activity modification. If nonoperative management fails, surgical joint arthroplasty or fusions are commonly performed.

CHAPTER 25

Hand and Wrist Bones

THE HAND
Congenital

During embryonic development, the hand forms from the limb bud. Congenital hand differences may occur due to disturbance in the development of the immature limb bud. Because other organ systems are developing at the same time with the limb bud, congenital hand abnormalities may be associated with disorders of other organ systems. Hence when evaluating congenital hand differences other musculoskeletal and systemic anomalies should be ruled out. Most congenital hand abnormalities are recognized at birth, some are diagnosed prenatally on ultrasound, and others become manifest later during childhood. Congenital hand abnormalities are classified into failure of formation (Fig. 25-1), failure of differentiation (Fig. 25-2), duplication (Fig. 25-3), overgrowth, undergrowth, amniotic constriction bands, and those associated with generalized abnormalities. Patients with congenital hand deformities should be referred to hand surgeons with expertise in pediatric hand surgery.

Trauma

Fractures are usually associated with swelling and subcutaneous ecchymosis. Skin integrity and the presence of any skeletal deformity should be evaluated. The osseous anatomy is easily palpated and areas of tenderness should be localized. Fractured bones are very tender to palpation. Range of motion of the joints adjacent to the fractured bone is often diminished due to pain. If there is any question about communication between a fracture and a nearby open wound, the fracture can be injected with saline or lidocaine. If the fluid leaks out through the wound, the fracture is considered open. The presence of fat droplets within the

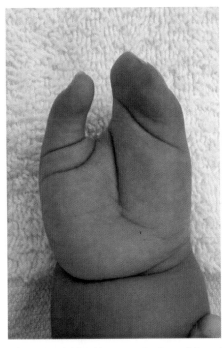

FIGURE 25-1 Congenital cleft hand is an example of many failure of formations. (Picture courtesy of Ghazi Rayan MD).

hemorrhagic blood is a better indication for the open nature of a fracture.

Fractures of long bones may angulate, rotate longitudinally, or shorten and lose opposition. Angular deformity is easy to detect (Fig. 25-4). The fingers should be examined while extended to assess for angular deformity either in the coronal or sagittal planes. The fingernails of the extended fingers can be viewed to assess for any rotational deformity. However, the best way to assess rotation is to view the fingertips end-on with the fingers flexed where rotation is often manifested as "scissoring," or digital overlap (Fig. 25-5). It is important to recognize that rotational deformity is best evaluated clinically, not radiographically.

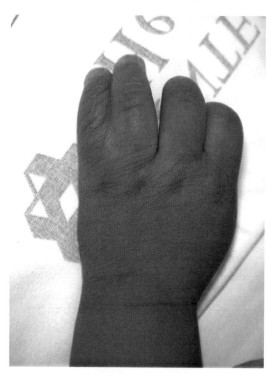

FIGURE 25-2 Congenital syndactyly is an example of many failure of differentiations. (Picture courtesy of Ghazi Rayan MD).

Radiographs may fail to reveal rotation that is obvious upon physical examination.

Active and passive joint range of motion should be measured. Loss of active motion can be due to pain, fracture, tenosynovitis, infection, or any pathology that inhibits the patient's desire for moving the joint. Loss of passive motion is due to inherent joint disease that limits mechanically its ability to move, such as contractures, arthritis, bony deformity, intraarticular fracture malunion, or chronic joint subluxation or dislocation.

Injuries to the radial and/or ulnar collateral ligaments (UCLs) of the interphalangeal joints and metacarpophalangeal (MP) joints

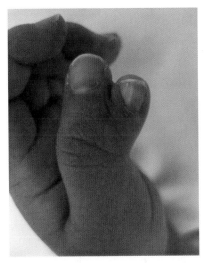

FIGURE 25-3 Congenital thumb polydactyly is an example of duplication. (Picture courtesy of Ghazi Rayan MD).

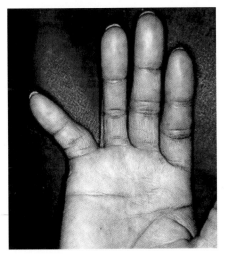

FIGURE 25-4 Angular deformity in the frontal plane due to P1 fracture malunion. (Picture courtesy of Ghazi Rayan MD).

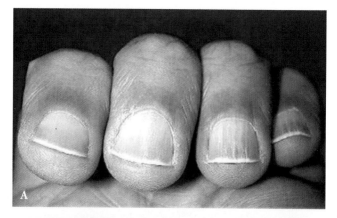

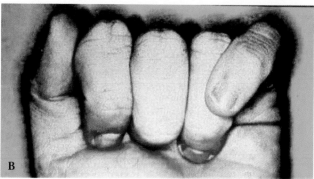

FIGURE 25-5 Viewed end-on with the fingers in flexion, the fingernails should demonstrate a slightly increasing inclination from the small finger to the index finger (**A**). Rotational deformity from a fractured or subluxed digit alters this normal digital cascade (**B**). (Pictures courtesy of Ghazi Rayan MD).

may be associated with avulsion fractures. Collateral ligament injuries often present as pain and swelling on the affected side of the joint. If fracture subluxation is present, the joint will deviate away from the side of the injured ligament.

Radiographs should be obtained for all traumatic injuries to rule out the presence of associated fractures. In cases of suspected phalangeal fractures and/or interphalangeal dislocations, it is important to acquire posteroanterior (PA), oblique, and true lateral radiographs of the injured finger and not to rely on radiographs of the hand. Radiographs of the hand do not provide appropriate detail of the individual digits and are best used for screening purposes or to evaluate the metacarpals. Radiographs of the hand may miss phalangeal fractures or subluxation that otherwise are evident on radiographs of the individual digits.

The thumb MP joint is prone to ligament injuries that can be associated with fractures. The UCL is often injured during falls where the thumb is caught by an object, such as a ski pole while skiing and hence it is known as "skier's thumb." The term "gamekeeper's thumb" is typically reserved for chronic UCL rupture that results from repetitive injury with subsequent instability. Associated bony avulsion from the base of the proximal phalanx may be present on radiographic examination. Acute UCL injuries have swelling and tenderness on the ulnar side of the thumb MP joint. Radial collateral ligament (RCL) injuries of the thumb are less common than ulnar. Associated bony avulsions are also less common with radial collateral ligament than UCL injuries.

The palmar plate of the proximal interphalangeal (PIP) joint, which prevents hyperextension, can also be injured. These are often associated with bony avulsion from the base of the P2. These are viewed on the X-ray as an intraarticular fragment from the volar base of P2.

THE WRIST

Examination of the wrist begins with observation for any swelling, bruising, or deformity. Any areas of tenderness should be elicited and localized. Distal radius fractures are very common (Fig. 25-6) and may be associated with wrist deformity and painful motion of radiocarpal joint and forearm motion. Radial-sided wrist pain with tenderness in the anatomic snuffbox following a fall on the outstretched hand is indicative of scaphoid fracture or scapholunate interosseous ligament injury until proven otherwise. The anatomic snuffbox, located between the first (abductor pollicis longus and extensor pollicis brevis) and third dorsal compartments (extensor pollicis longus), is best seen

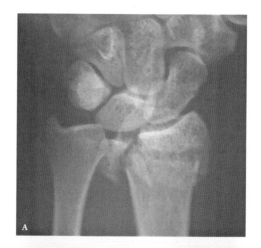

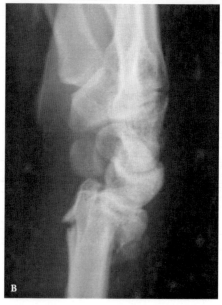

FIGURE 25-6 X-ray PA (**A**) and lateral (**B**) views of an intraarticular distal radius fracture.

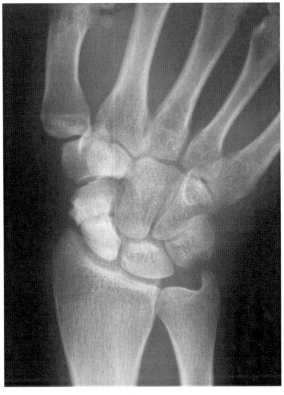

FIGURE 25-7 PA elongation (wrist ulnar deviation) X-ray view showing scaphoid fracture nonunion.

by having the patient extend the thumb. Scaphoid fracture is not readily visualized on radiographs except with certain special elongation views (Fig. 25-7).

The hook of the hamate (hamulus) is another osseous carpal structure whose fracture is often not visible on standard radiographs. The hamulus may fracture following a fall, but more commonly is fractured during racquet sports, such as tennis or from golfing. To palpate the hamulus, the examiner places his thumb interphalangeal joint on the pisiform bone, at the distal extent of the flexor carpi ulnaris tendon so that the tip of the thumb points at a 45° angle toward the web space between the patient's thumb and index fingers. The examiner's thumb tip will rest on the hamulus. If that area is tender following a traumatic episode, hamulus fracture should be suspected.

HAND AND WRIST

Tumors

Bony tumors of the hand and wrist may be benign or malignant. Benign tumors are much more common. Tumors should be inspected for their exact location and any overlying skin changes. Palpation should determine tenderness, consistency, and mobility of the mass. The most common benign bony tumor of the hand is enchondroma.

Infection

Infections of the bony structures of the hand and wrist may be acute or chronic and called osteomyelitis. Examination should identify the location of associate overlying cellulitis, the presence of which should be outlined with a marker for future follow up. A localized tenderness or fluctuant mass is suggestive of underlying abscess. Osteomyelitis is a serious disease that may jeopardize the affected part if not treated appropriately. Radiographic examination is diagnostic. The clinician should have a high index of suspicion for osteomyelitis following open fractures complicated by chronic pain, swelling, or drainage.

Treatment

Non-displaced fractures of the hand and wrist are usually treated nonoperatively, with immobilization until they are healed enough to permit joint range of motion. Reducible displaced fractures are treated with manipulation in order to achieve closed anatomical reduction. If the fracture is stable following closed reduction, cast immobilization is utilized in the reduced position. If the fracture is unstable, percutaneous pin fixation is often used. If the fracture is not reducible by closed means, then open reduction with internal fixation is usually required.

Tumors are often excised if painful and increasing in size. Infections that involve the bone or abscess formation should be surgically drained and debrided along with intravenous antibiotics.

Amputations

The indications for replantation have changed in the last several years and become more limited. With some exceptions, hand function following single finger amputations such as the index in adults will be superior with acceptance of the loss of the part than following replantation. Replantation is a major undertaking that requires hospitalization and may result in delayed return to work, residual pain, decreased sensibility, cold intolerance, stiffness, and dysfunction of the replanted part. All this may greatly decrease the function of the entire hand that would have remained more functional had the replantation not been performed.

Current indications for replantation include sharp guillotine amputation of the thumb, as this is the most important digit in the hand, and the thumb does not require great motion to be functional. A stiff thumb that opposes against the fingers can be highly functional, as opposed to the fingers that require substantial motion to be functional. Multiple digital amputations should be replanted, as should any digit in a child, who is less prone to joint stiffness and tendinous scarring than adults. Amputations through the hand itself or proximal to the hand should also be replanted, due to the substantial loss of function that would otherwise ensue. In the fingers the best results are achieved for amputations distal to the PIP joint, as these result in minimal PIP joint stiffness. The limit of most microsurgical vascular repairs is 0.5 mm, which is the size of the digital artery at the level of the distal interphalangeal joint in an adult and at the PIP joint in a child. In adults, this essentially limits the optimal indications for replantation for sharp amputations through the distal aspect of the middle phalanx. Replantations for amputations through zone II of the finger (proximal to the flexor digitorum superficialis insertion, where both flexor tendons are within the flexor sheath) have little functional benefit to the hand, because of the prolonged time away from work and substantial stiffness, which often impairs overall hand function. The exception to this is the thumb, where there is only one flexor tendon, and stiffness is not very dysfunctional.

In order to be suitable for replantation an amputated digit needs to have tidy margins. Digits with multi-level injury such as crush and avulsions are not suitable for replantation. Patients with multiple medical problems are challenging for long surgery and those with cardiac disease or who refuse to stop smoking are not candidates for replantation. Patients with self-inflicted amputations should not undergo replantation, as 95% will re-amputate the part within 6 months.

Acute care of the amputated part is of paramount importance. During transportation to a replantation center the part should be wrapped in a saline-moistened gauze and sealed in a plastic bag. The plastic bag should be placed on ice. The amputated part itself should never be directly placed on ice, as this will lead to frostbite and vessel damage. For similar reasons, dry ice should never be used. The amputated part should not be immersed in water, which also damages its tissues.

The warm ischemic time for a digit, which does not contain muscle (muscle is very metabolically active and undergoes necrosis most readily) should be 6 hours or less. For a digit, in some circumstances up to 24 hours of cold ischemia time, can be tolerated. For amputations proximal to the carpus, which contain muscle, warm ischemia time should be less than 3 hours, to avoid muscle necrosis, which precludes safe and effective replantation.

Key to Abbreviations in the Text

ADM	abductor digiti minimi
AdP	adductor pollicis
ADQ	abductor digit quinti
AIN	anterior interosseus nerve
APB	abductor pollicis brevis
APL	abductor pollicis longus
BCC	basal cell carcinoma
CMC	carpometacarpal
CTS	carpal tunnel syndrome
DD	Dupuytren disease
DIC	dorsal intercarpal
DISI	dorsal intercalated segment instability
DIP	distal interphalangeal
DRC	dorsal radiocarpal
DRUJ	distal radioulnar joint
DVT	deep venous thrombosis
ECRB	extensor carpi radialis brevis
ECRL	extensor carpi radialis longus
ECU	extensor carpi ulnaris
EDC	extensor digitorum communis
EDM	extensor digiti minimi (quinti)

EIP	extensor indicis proprius
EPB	extensor pollicis brevis
EPL	extensor pollicis longus
FCR	flexor carpi radialis
FDP	flexor digitorum profundus
FDQ	flexor digiti quinti (minimi)
FDS	flexor digitorum superficialis
FPB	flexor pollicis brevis
FPL	flexor pollicis longus
IP	interphalangeal
IPPL	interpalmar plate ligament
LT	lunotriquetral
LTIL	lunotriquetral interosseous ligament
MP	metacarpophalangeal
MPJ	metacarpophalangeal joint
MRI	magnetic resonance imaging
NV	neurovascular
ODM	opponens digiti minimi
ODQ	opponens digiti quinti
OP	opponens pollicis
P1	proximal phalanx
P2	middle phalanx
P3	distal phalanx
PA	posteroanterior
PB	palmaris brevis
PIN	posterior interosseus nerve
PIP	proximal interphalangeal
PL	palmaris longus

PQ	pronator quadrates
PT	pronator teres
PVR	pulse volume recording
RA	rheumatoid arthritis
RCL	radial collateral ligament
ROM	range of motion
SCC	squamous cell carcinoma
SL	scapholunate
SLAC	scapholunate advanced collapse
SLIL	scapholunate interosseous ligament
TCL	transverse carpal ligament
TFCC	triangular fibrocartilage complex
TLPA	transverse ligament of the palmar aponeurosis
TM	trapeziometacarpal
UCL	ulnar collateral ligament
VISI	volar intercalated segment instability

Suggested Book Readings

American Society for Surgery of the Hand. *The First Fifty Years.* New York, Edinburgh, London, Madrid, Melbourne, San Francisco, Tokyo: Churchill Livingstone; 1995.

Berger R, Weiss A-Peter, eds. *Hand Surgery.* Philadelphia: Lippincott Williams & Wilkins; 2004.

Boyes JH, eds. *On the Shoulders of Giants, Notable Names in Hand Surgery.* Philadelphia, PA: J.B. Lippincott, 1976.

Budoff JE, ed. *Fractures of the Upper Extremity: A Masters Skills Publication.* American Society for Surgery of the Hand; 2008.

Bunnell S, ed. *Surgery of the Hand.* Philadelphia, PA: J. B. Lippincott; 1948.

Burns T, Breathnach S, Cox N, Griffith C, eds. *Rook's Textbook of Dermatology,* 7th ed. Malden: Blackwell Publishers; 2004.

Doyle J, Botte M, eds. Surgical Anatomy of the Hand and Upper Extremity. Philadelphia: Lippincott Williams & Wilkins; 2003.

Gelberman RH, ed. *Master Techniques in Orthopaedic Surgery: The Wrist.* Philadelphia: Lippincott Williams & Wilkins; 2009.

Hammert W, Calfee R, Bozentka D, Boyer M, eds. *Manual of Hand Surgery.* American Society for Surgery of the Hand; 2010.

Kaplan EB, ed. *Functional and surgical anatomy of the hand.* 2nd ed. Philadelphia, PA: J. B. Lippincott; 1965.

Mathes S, Hentz V, eds. *Plastic Surgery,* 2nd ed. Philadelphia: Elsevier; 2006.

Meals R. *The Hand Owner's Manual.* virtualbookworm.com, 2008.

Rayan GM, ed. *Nerve Compression Syndromes – Hand Clinics.* Philadelphia: WB Saunders; 1992.

Rayan GM, Chung KC, eds. *Flap Reconstruction of the Upper Extremity: A Masters Skills Presentation.* Chicago, IL: American Society for Surgery of the Hand; 2009.

Robinson JK, Hanke CW, Siegel DM, Fratila A, eds. *Surgery of the Skin: Procedural Dermatology.* 2nd ed. Philadelphia,. PA: Elsevier; 2010.

Slutsky D, ed. *Upper Extremity Nerve Repair – Tips and Techniques. Chicago:* American Society for Surgery of the Hand; 2008.

Spinner M, ed. *Kaplan's Functional and Surgical Anatomy of the Hand.* 3rd ed. Philadelphia, PA: J.B. Lippincott; 1984.

Standring S, ed. *Gray's Anatomy: The Anatomical Basis of Clinical Practice,* 40th ed. London: Churchill Livingstone/Elsevier; 2008.

Trumble T, Budoff JE, eds. *Hand Surgery Update 4. Chicago: American Society for Surgery of the Hand*; 2007.

Trumble T, Rayan GM, Budoff JE, Baratz ME, eds. *Principles of Hand Surgery and Therapy.* 2nd ed. Philadelphia, PA: Saunders Elsevier; 2009.

Wiesel S, ed. *Operative Techniques in Orthopedic Surgery*. Philadelphia: Lippincott Williams & Wilkins. 2010.

Wolfe SW, Hotchkiss RN, Pedersen WC, Kozin SH, eds. *Green's Operative Hand Surgery*. 6th ed. Philadelphia, PA: Elsevier Churchill Livingstone; 2011.

Yu H-L, Chase RA, Strauch B, eds. *Atlas of Hand Anatomy and Clinical Implications*. St Louis, MO: Mosby; 2003.

Zook EG Brrown R, eds. *The Perionychium – Hand Clinics*. Philadelphia: WB Saunders; 2002.

Index

NOTE: Page numbers followed by 'f' indicate figures.